Fat Oppression around the World

This book offers cutting-edge, intersectional, and interdisciplinary research in the blossoming field of fat studies. The aim is to generate discussion about the complexity of fat oppression as a phenomenon and social force that permeates interactions both at an institutional and interpersonal level, impacting the lived experiences of fat people.

Each chapter has been carefully selected to create a space to showcase the engaging intersectional and interdisciplinary fat-studies scholarship that is taking place globally. This engaging book will take the reader around the world by examining: weight-loss classes in Ireland, Jamaican women's views of health and fatness, the difficulties of immigrating while fat to New Zealand, fat activism in Finnish media, being fat and pregnant in Australia, a girls' camp in the United States, and the experiences of fat hatred felt by queer fat women in Canada. This book will inspire fat-studies scholars globally to incorporate intersectional approaches and qualitative methods in future work.

The chapters in this book were originally published in *Fat Studies: An Interdisciplinary Journal of Body Weight and Society*.

Ariane Prohaska is Associate Professor of Sociology in the Department of Criminology and Criminal Justice at the University of Alabama. Her research interests include gender, bodies, fat studies, and disaster sociology. She has recently published in *Fat Studies*, *Critical Policy Studies*, and *International Journal of Mass Emergencies and Disasters*.

Jeannine A. Gailey is Professor of Sociology at Texas Christian University. She studies gender, bodies, fat studies, and sexualities. Her recent research has appeared in *Fat Studies*, *Feminism & Psychology*, and *Qualitative Research*. Her monograph, *The Hyper(in)visible Fat Woman*, was published in 2014.

Fat Oppression around the World

Intersectional, Interdisciplinary, and
Methodological Innovations

Edited by
Ariane Prohaska and Jeannine A. Gailey

Routledge
Taylor & Francis Group

LONDON AND NEW YORK

First published 2022
by Routledge
2 Park Square, Milton Park, Abingdon, Oxon OX14 4RN

and by Routledge
605 Third Avenue, New York, NY 10158

Routledge is an imprint of the Taylor & Francis Group, an informa business
Introduction, Chapters 1–4, 6 and 7 © 2022 Taylor & Francis

Chapter 5 © 2019 Jennifer Lee. Originally published as Open Access.

British Library Cataloguing in Publication Data
A catalogue record for this book is available from the British Library

ISBN: 978-0-367-74664-3 (hbk)
ISBN: 978-0-367-74665-0 (pbk)
ISBN: 978-1-003-15897-4 (ebk)

Typeset in Minion Pro
by Newgen Publishing UK

Publisher's Note
The publisher accepts responsibility for any inconsistencies that may have arisen during the conversion of this book from journal articles to book chapters, namely the inclusion of journal terminology.

Disclaimer
Every effort has been made to contact copyright holders for their permission to reprint material in this book. The publishers would be grateful to hear from any copyright holder who is not here acknowledged and will undertake to rectify any errors or omissions in future editions of this book.

Contents

Citation Information

The following chapters were originally published in two issues of *Fat Studies: An Interdisciplinary Journal of Body Weight and Society*. When citing this material, please use the original citations and page numbering for each article, as follows:

Introduction
Theorizing fat oppression: Intersectional approaches and methodological innovations
Ariane Prohaska and Jeannine A. Gailey
Fat Studies, volume 8, issue 1 (2019), pp. 1–9

Chapter 1
Crafting weight stigma in slimming classes: A case study in Ireland
Jacqueline O'Toole
Fat Studies, volume 8, issue 1 (2019), pp. 10–24

Chapter 2
Understanding fatness: Jamaican women's constructions of health
Claudia Barned and Kieran O'Doherty
Fat Studies, volume 8, issue 1 (2019), pp. 25–43

Chapter 3
Frozen: A fat tale of immigration
Cat Pausé
Fat Studies, volume 8, issue 1 (2019), pp. 44–59

Chapter 4
Can ambivalence hold potential for fat activism? An analysis of conflicting discourses on fatness in the Finnish column series Jenny's Life Change
Anna Puhakka
Fat Studies, volume 8, issue 1 (2019), pp. 60–74

For any permission-related enquiries please visit:
www.tandfonline.com/page/help/permissions

Notes on Contributors

Claudia Barned, Pragmatic Health Ethics Research Unit, Institut de recherches cliniques de Montréal, Montréal, Quebec, Canada.

Trisha L. Crawshaw, Department of Sociology, Southern Illinois University, Carbondale, USA.

Jeannine A. Gailey, Department of Sociology and Anthropology, Texas Christian University, Fort Worth, Texas, USA.

Crystal Kotow, PhD, Centre for Academic Excellence, St. Clair College, Windsor, ON, Canada.

Jennifer Lee, Institute for Health and Sport, Victoria University, Melbourne, Australia.

Emma Lind, Gender, Sexuality, and Women's Studies, Okanagan College, Kelowna BC, Canada.

Kieran O'Doherty, Department of Psychology, University of Guelph, Guelph, Ontario, Canada.

Jacqueline O'Toole, Department of Social Sciences, Institute of Technology, Sligo, Republic of Ireland.

Cat Pausé, Institute of Education, College of Humanities and Social Sciences, Massey University, Palmerston North, New Zealand.

Ariane Prohaska, Department of Criminology and Criminal Justice, University of Alabama, Tuscaloosa, Alabama, USA.

Anna Puhakka, Department of Social Sciences and Philosophy, University of Jyväskylä, Jyväskylä, Finland.

Carla Rice, College of Social & Applied Human Sciences, University of Guelph, Guelph ON, Canada.

Jen Rinaldi, Legal Studies, University of Ontario Institute of Technology, Oshawa ON, Canada.

Theorizing fat oppression: Intersectional approaches and methodological innovations

Ariane Prohaska and Jeannine A. Gailey

About fifteen years ago, as PhD students in sociology, we discovered a little-known practice often referred to as "hogging." Hogging occurs when some men, usually college-aged or in the military, seek out fat women as sexual partners for one of two reasons: (1) they think that fat women are desperate and easy to lure into sexual favors, or (2) they are trying to win a bet with their friends about who can "take home" (and have sex with) the largest woman (see Gailey and Prohaska 2006; Prohaska and Gailey 2009, 2010). The phenomenon of hogging is deeply rooted in both culturally sanctioned misogyny and stereotypes that equate beauty and sexual attractiveness with thinness.

When we began our research on hogging in 2004, we were unaware of the emerging field of fat studies. Some fifteen years later, the multidisciplinary and interdisciplinary field has substantially grown. For example, fat studies now has its own journal; numerous monographs; edited collections of research about the societal treatment of fat and how that impacts the lives of people of size; and popular sessions at international, national, and regional scholarly meetings. In our introduction to this collection of scholarship about fat oppression, we discuss the meaning of oppression, both generally and within fat studies, and review the literature on how cultural definitions of fat affect the experiences of people who are fat at multiple levels of analysis. We highlight how the articles selected for this issue enrich the theoretical and empirical understanding of fat oppression, giving special attention to research that highlights how fatness intersects with other social identities, such as race, gender, sexualities, age, and so forth.

Oppression

From a sociological perspective, *oppression* refers to the systemic constraints placed on marginalized and underprivileged groups that are institutionalized via the values, norms, laws, and institutions in a society (Young 1990). Systemic oppression results in unequal life chances (opportunities) and social outcomes for marginalized groups. The most pernicious and overt forms of oppression are institutional barriers, such as discrimination in education, the workplace, the media, and health care. Less obvious is symbolic oppression (Crandall 1994), which occurs when marginalized groups are assumed to lack values deemed crucial to society. For example, racial oppression in the United States is exacerbated by commonly held beliefs that people of color—namely, those who identify as African American or Black—do not ascribe to the values of hard work, self-reliance, and motivation (Sears 1988). Similarly, people who are fat are often assumed to be lazy, irresponsible, and gluttonous (Schwartz et al. 2006).

One of the key aspects of oppression is that it is often "invisible" (Frye 1983), and thus oppressed people are frequently blamed for the discrimination and mistreatment they receive, creating a vicious cycle that reinforces oppression and can lead to the oppressed group internalizing dominant ideologies and even feeling responsible for their own marginalization (Collins 1990). If cultural norms about the group become internalized, members of the marginalized group are more likely to face negative consequences, particularly with regard to economic and psychological well-being. While oppression based on race, class, gender, sexuality, and age has been studied for a few decades, the introduction of fat studies to the academy, particularly *The Fat Studies Reader* (Rothblum and Solovay 2009) and the journal *Fat Studies*, created an intellectual space for theoretical and empirical scholarship on people who are fat and their status as an oppressed group.

Oppression of fat people

Eller (2014) writes that "Fat people suffer, and they suffer in virtue of being fat" (220). The oppression of people who are fat is systematic and systemic, as negative ideologies about fat pervade societal institutions. The classification of "obesity" as "epidemic" in medicine and as a disease by the American Medical Association resulted in the labeling of fat as a social problem and pathological condition that needs to be remedied. These characterizations have led to heightened attention on people who are fat not only from medical professionals but also from academics, the media, the diet industry, and myriad other institutions in society (e.g., Boero 2013; Gailey 2014). What Crandall (1994) terms the symbolic prejudice of fat consists of "beliefs and values that reflect self-determination and the Puritan work ethic" (883). The rhetoric surrounding the "obesity epidemic" emphasizes individual responsibility, leading to the supposition that people are fat because they eat too much, exercise too little, and are resistant to "treatments" for their "problems" (e.g., Lupton 2014). These beliefs result in the shaming and blaming of fat people, and research has shown that people who are fat are frequently assumed to be lazy, unmotivated, and socially inferior (Schwartz et al. 2006). Moreover, this implicit bias against people who are fat is developed early in life (Skinner et al. 2017).

Gailey (2014) argues that people who are fat, as well as other marginalized groups, experience "hyper(in)visibility," which renders their bodies and behaviors constantly policed, while their oppression as a group is ignored. The labeling of "obesity" as a social problem persists despite scholarly evidence that shows that much of the attention on "obesity" is overstated and hyperbolic (see, for instance, Flegal et al. 2005, 2013; Gard and Wright 2005; Wright and

Harwood 2009). When circulated by the media, this misinformation can lead to interpersonal and institutional violence against fat people (see Rothblum 1999; Saguy and Almeling 2008). In this book, O'Toole's analysis of slimming classes in Ireland reveals that the reliance on the "obesity epidemic" narrative in fitness culture, which focuses on weight loss rather than health, again problematizes fat bodies. In essence, slimming classes focus on the problems with fat and the need for individuals to lose weight, regardless of their health status. The slimming classes that O'Toole studied comprise the largest for-profit weight-loss program in the country. Her data indicate that these slimming classes are not only popular but also help shape the public perception that fat is unhealthy and unattractive.

The medical establishment, politicians, and the media have pathologized "obesity" and labeled it a disease (Kwan and Graves 2013; Saguy and Almeling 2008). Barned and O'Doherty's chapter about the intersection of race, body size, and health in Jamaica examines the cultural norms surrounding fat in a non-White, non-North American context, offering an account of health that subverts the oppressive "obesity epidemic" discourse. They argue that a slim-thick healthy body discourse, which emerged in their study, is one such discourse that attends to the fat acceptance ideology. Fat acceptance activists challenge the medical and public health paradigm that fat is unhealthy or unattractive. According to this alternative framework, fat is beautiful, healthy, a form of natural bodily diversity, and the basis for civil rights claims (Saguy 2013). Moreover, fat acceptance advocates challenge the dominant frame by embracing the word "fat" as a basis of identity. In other words, using the word "fat" as an identity marker serves to challenge the cultural belief that being fat is the "worst quality a person can have."

On an institutional level, the rhetoric surrounding the "obesity epidemic" translates into discrimination against fat people. According to National Association to Advance Fat Acceptance (2014), size discrimination occurs as frequently as racial discrimination and has increased since the late 1990s. In the workplace, people who are fat are often denied access to promotions and higher wages due to their size (Fikkan and Rothblum 2005; Gapinski, Schwartz, and Brownell 2006). In education, "obesity" paradigms take prevalence in health, medical, and physical education (O'Brien, Hunter, and Banks 2007; Sykes and McPhail 2008), and professors who are fat frequently confront discrimination in their classrooms (Escalera 2009).

In television and film, people who are fat are often portrayed negatively (Himes and Thompson 2007; Hussin, Frazier, and Thompson 2011; Mendoza 2009; Sender and Sullivan 2008). Fat characters are typically the targets of fatphobic humor, and makeover shows seek to "fix" fat people through weight loss. For example, the hit television show *The Biggest Loser* is broadcast in over 90 countries and features contestants who compete to lose the most weight through drastic diet changes and exercise with the assistance of a personal trainer. Some of the contestants reportedly have maintained weight loss, but others have come forward stating that the show promotes unhealthy weight loss through questionable means.[1] In addition to allegedly promoting unrealistic weight loss, the show perpetuates the larger societal view that losing a significant amount of weight is achievable through hard work—as if fat and laziness are interrelated (Gailey 2014).

People of size are also discriminated against in the legal system. In the courtroom, people who are fat are presumed guilty more than their thin counterparts (Beety 2012). Crime victims who are fat are classified as pitiful and helpless because of their size or, at least for women, not perceived as believable victims of intimate partner violence or sexual assault because they do not fit the stereotype of a "typical" (thin or attractive) victim. Relatedly, many public spaces are inaccessible or unaccommodating to fat people, including airplanes (Huff 2009), other forms of public transportation, restaurants, doctors' offices, and so forth (Gailey 2014; Owen 2012). Moreover, fat is not a protected class under discrimination laws in most locations in the world (e.g., Jones 2012; Rothblum 2012). Cat Pausé's chapter discusses the difficulties she faced obtaining a permanent work visa in New Zealand because of her weight. In other words, New Zealand's immigration department actively excludes those whose bodies are deemed fat from receiving work visas because of the assumed burden that fat bodies will place on New Zealand's government sponsored health-care system.

Interpersonally, fat women are sanctioned and often mistreated in relationships. Research indicates that fat women are less likely than their thin counterparts to be labeled as desirable relationship or sexual partners (e.g., Chen and Brown 2005; Gailey 2012; Gimlin 2002; Swami, Steadman, and Tovee 2009). Within intimate relationships, fat women are just as likely as thinner women to experience physical, sexual, and emotional abuse (e.g., Fabrizio 2014; Gailey 2014, 2012; Gailey and Prohaska 2006; Prohaska and Gailey 2010, 2009; Royce 2009). And fat children and adolescents are more likely to be bullied than their thin peers (Weinstock and Krehbiel 2009).

Institutional and interpersonal fat oppression ultimately becomes internalized by fat people resulting in myriad negative consequences. Despite the fact that the fat acceptance movement has fostered feelings of fat pride for some (Gailey 2014, 2012), the impact of stigma can lead to feelings of shame, isolation, lower self-esteem, poor body image, and an increased risk of other mental health issues and some medical conditions compared to their thin counterparts (e.g., Carr and Friedman 2005; Davidson et al. 2008; Miller and Downey 1999; O'Dea 2006). Indeed, fat shaming under the guise of concern for health does not lead to weight loss or to an increase in activities associated with losing weight (Davidson et al. 2008; Gailey 2014; Puhl, Moss-Racusin, and Schwartz 2007; Schafer and Ferraro 2011; Sutin and Terracciano 2013).

Four chapters in this book examine how institutional beliefs and practices impact the lived experiences of fat people. Lee's autoethnography highlights both the intersections of pregnancy, fatness, and motherhood and the impact of institutional discrimination (in this case, the institution of medicine) on her experiences of pregnancy, childbirth, and motherhood. Puhakka's chapter reveals the mixed messages conveyed by a Finnish weight-loss campaign called the Scale Rebellion that intended to address fatness through body positivity and fat activism. Results from her content analysis indicates that the message of the Scale Rebellion was often mixed and ambiguous in nature. The main figure of the campaign, Jenny, often discussed her desire to lose weight, contributing to mixed messages regarding fatness and body positivity. Puhakka argues that ambivalence present in the messages is a product of the stigmatized nature of fatness in the culture rather than a representation that an activist is a sell-out or fake. Similarly, Crawshaw's research on "Girl's Rock" camp, a self-proclaimed "body positive" space for young women, identifies the conflicting messages girls receive about fat bodies within this space and how they negotiate these messages with their feelings about their own bodies via "resistance work." Rinaldi, Rice, Kotow, and Lind's chapter also focuses on the internalization of fatphobia. The authors use the lenses of affect theory and intersectionality-as-assemblage theory to guide their interviews with queer and trans individuals about their experiences of fatmisia (i.e. fat hatred) in health care, in public transportation, and at exercise facilities.

The institutional, interpersonal, and internalized oppression that fat people experience intersects with other types of oppression based on race, class, gender, ability, sexuality, and nation, among other social statuses (for more on intersectionality, see Cho, Crenshaw, and McCall 2013; Crenshaw 1991; Collins 1990; Pausé 2014). Although there are several phenomenal pieces of fat studies research that theorize how fat interacts with other dimensions of oppression (some notable examples include Whitesel's (2017) examination of how fat Black Americans experience negative interactions with police, and Sojka and Sanchez's (2019) call for the inclusion of trans masculine and intersex individuals in fat studies work on reproductive health care), there is more work to be done. It is imperative to examine these relationships because of the qualitatively different ways that women, people of color, LGBTQ+, the working class and poor, differently abled, and non-Western and/or non-North American people, among others, experience fatness within particular legal and cultural contexts, which is why were deliberate in choosing manuscripts for this collection that examine the intersections between fat and other social identity markers.

Conclusion

We hope that the chapters in this book generate further discussion about the complexity of fat oppression as a phenomenon and social force that permeates our interactions institutionally and interpersonally. As we selected manuscripts for our special issues in the *Fat Studies Journal*, we heeded the advice of Cat Pausé (2014), urging those who are writing, researching, or publishing fat studies work to "create spaces that allow for intersectional scholarship, and to be willing to sit at a variety of tables" (84). Although the scholarship that follows cannot account for the experiences of all people of size, we trust that *Fat Studies* has created a space at the table for scholars who employ an intersectional lens. In addition, as feminists in the field of sociology, we are painfully aware that qualitative methodologies are frequently subordinated, so we thought it was important to select manuscripts that utilize these underrepresented methodologies for an issue on oppression. Moreover, given that we were interested in showcasing research that employs an intersectional approach, qualitative research methods seemed to be the natural fit. It is our hope that this collection will inspire fat studies scholars to incorporate intersectional approaches and qualitative methods in future work.

Finally, we would like to thank the authors who responded to our call for abstracts about fat oppression. We are encouraged that so many scholars are entering the field of fat studies. We are especially grateful to the reviewers and to Esther Rothblum for her guidance as we navigated journal editorship for the first time, and to Robinson Raju, who helped us through the editing process of this book. Lastly, we want to thank Hannah Taylor for her editorial support.

Note

1. www.huffingtonpost.com/2009/11/25/biggest-loser-contestants_n_370538.html   (accessed April 10, 2010).

References

Beety, V. 2012. "Criminality and Corpulence: Weight Bias in the Courtroom." *Seattle Journal for Social Justice* 11 (2):523–24.

Boero, N. 2013. "Obesity in the Media: Social Science Weighs In." *Critical Public Health* 23 (3):371–80. doi:10.1080/09581596.2013.783686.

Carr, D., and M.A. Friedman. 2005. "Is Obesity Stigmatizing? Body Weight, Perceived Discrimination, and Psychological Well-Being in the United States." *Journal of Health and Social Behavior* 46 (3):244–59. doi:10.1177/002214650504600303.

Chen, E., and M. Brown. 2005. "Obesity Stigma in Sexual Relationships." *Obesity Research* 13 (8):1393–97. doi:10.1038/oby.2005.168.

Cho, S., K. W. Crenshaw, and L. McCall. 2013. "Toward a Field of Intersectionality Studies: Theory, Applications, and Praxis." *Signs: Journal of Women in Culture and Society* 38 (4):785–810. doi:10.1086/669608.

Collins, P. H. 1990. *Black Feminist Thought: Knowledge, Consciousness, and the Politics of Empowerment.* NY: Routledge.

Crandall, C. 1994. "Prejudice against Fat People: Ideology and Self-Interest." *Journal of Personality and Social Psychology* 66 (5):882–94.

Crenshaw, K. 1991. "Mapping the Margins: Intersectionality, Identity Politics, and Violence against Women of Color." *Stanford Law Review* 43 (6):1241–99. doi:10.2307/1229039.

Davidson, K. K., D. L. Schmalz, L. M. Young, and L. L. Birch. 2008. "Overweight Girls Who Internalize Fat Stereotypes Report Low Psychological Well-Being." *Obesity* 16 (S2):30–38. doi:10.1038/oby.2008.451.

Eller, G.M. 2014. "On Fat Oppression." *Kennedy Institute of Ethics Journal* 24 (3):219–45.

Escalera, E. A. 2009. "Stigma Threat and the Fat Professor: Reducing Student Prejudice in the Classroom." In *The Fat Studies Reader*, Eds. E. Rothblum and S. Solovay, 205–12. New York, NY: New York University Press.

Fabrizio, M. 2014. "Abundantly Invisible: Fat Oppression as a Framework for Sexual Violence against Women." *Spaces Between: an Undergraduate Feminist Journal* 2:1–14.

Fikkan, J., and E. Rothblum. 2005. "Weight Bias in Employment." In *Weight Bias: Nature, Consequences, and Remedies*, Eds. K. D. Brownell, R. M. Puhl, M. B. Schwartz, and L. Rudd, 15–28. New York, NY: Guilford Publications.

Flegal, K. M., B. I. Graubard, D. F. Williamson, and M. H. Gail. 2005. "Excess Deaths Associated with Overweight, Underweight, and Obesity." *JAMA* 293:1861–67. doi: 10.1001/jama.293.15.1861.

Flegal, K. M., B. K. Kit, H. Orbana, and B. I. Graubard. 2013. "Association of All-Cause Mortality with Overweight and Obesity Using Standard Body Mass Index Categories: A Systematic Review and Meta-Analysis." *JAMA* 309:71–82. doi: 10.1001/jama.2012.113905.

Frye, M. 1983. *The Politics of Reality*. Freedom, CA: Crossing.

Gailey, J. A. 2012. "Fat Shame to Fat Pride: Fat Women's Sexual and Dating Experiences." *Fat Studies* 1 (1):114–27. doi:10.1080/21604851.2012.631113.

Gailey, J. A. 2014. *The Hyper(In)Visible Fat Woman*. New York, NY: Palgrave Macmillan.

Gailey, J. A., and A. Prohaska. 2006. "Knocking of a Fat Girl: An Exploration of Deviance, Male Sexuality, and Neutralizations." *Deviant Behavior* 27 (1):31–46. doi:10.1080/016396290968353.

Gapinski, K. D., M. B. Schwartz, and K. D. Brownell. 2006. "Can Television Change Anti-Fat Attitudes and Behavior?" *Journal of Applied Biobehavioral Research* 11 (1):1–28. doi:10.1111/j.1751-9861.2006.tb00017.x.

Gard, M., and J. Wright. 2005. *The Obesity Epidemic: Science, Morality, and Ideology*. New York, NY: Routledge.

Gimlin, D. 2002. *Body Work: Beauty and Self-Image in American Culture*. Berkeley: University of California Press.

Himes, S. M., and J. K. Thompson. 2007. "Fat Stigmatization in Television Shows and Movies: A Content Analysis." *Obesity* 15 (3):712–18. doi:10.1038/oby.2007.635.

Huff, J. L. 2009. "Access to the Sky: Airplane Seats and Fat Bodies as Contested Spaces." In *The Fat Studies Reader*, Eds. E. Rothblum and S. Solovay, 176–86. New York, NY: New York University Press.

Hussin, M., S. Frazier, and J. K. Thompson. 2011. "Fat Stigmatization on YouTube: A Content Analysis." *Body Image* 8 (1):90–92. doi:10.1016/j.bodyim.2010.10.003.

Jones, L. E. 2012. "The Framing of Fat: Narratives of Health and Disability in Fat Discrimination Legislation." *New York University Law Review* 87 (6):1996–2039.

Kwan, S., and J. Graves. 2013. *Framing Fat: Competing Constructions in Contemporary Culture*. New Brunswick, NJ: Rutgers University Press.

Lupton, D. 2014. "The Pedagogy of Disgust: The Ethical, Moral and Political Implications of Using Disgust in Public Health Campaigns." *Critical Public Health* 25 (1):1–11.

Mendoza, K. 2009. "Seeing through the Layers: Fat Suits and Thin Bodies in *the Nutty Professor* and *Shallow Hal*." In *The Fat Studies Reader*, Eds. E. Rothblum and S. Solovay, 280–88. New York, NY: New York University Press.

Miller, C. T., and K. T. Downey. 1999. "A Meta-Analysis of Heavyweight and Self-Esteem." *Personality and Social Psychology Review* 3 (1):68–84. doi:10.1207/s15327957pspr0301_4.

National Association to Advance Fat Acceptance (2014). Facts on Size Discrimination. www.naafaonline.com/dev2/assets/documents/naafa_FactSheet_v17_screen.pdf. Accessed July 5, 2018.

O'Brien, K.S., J.A. Hunter, and M. Banks. 2007. "Implicit Anti-Fat Bias in Physical Educators: Physical Attributes, Ideology and Socialization." *International Journal of Obesity 31* 31:308–14. doi: 10.1038/sj.ijo.0803398.

O'Dea, J. A. 2006. "Self-Concept, Self-Esteem and Body Weight in Adolescent Females: A Three Year Longitudinal Study." *Journal of Health Psychology* 11 (4):599–611. doi:10.1177/1359105306065020.

Owen, L. 2012. "Living Fat in a Thin-Centric World: Effects of Spatial Discrimination on Fat Bodies and Selves." *Feminism & Psychology* 22 (3):290–306. doi:10.1177/0959353512445360.

Pausé, C. J. 2014. "X-Static Process: Intersectionality within the Field of Fat Studies." *Fat Studies: an Interdisciplinary Journal of Body Weight and Society* 3 (2):80–85. doi:10.1080/21604851.2014.889487.

Prohaska, A., and J. A. Gailey. 2009. "Fat Women as Easy Targets: Achieving Masculinity through Hogging." In *The Fat Studies Reader*, Eds. E. Rothblum and S. Solovay, 158–66. New York, NY: New York University Press.

Prohaska, A., and J. A. Gailey. 2010. "Achieving Masculinity through Sexual Predation: The Case of Hogging." *Journal of Gender Studies* 19 (1):13–25. doi:10.1080/09589230903525411.

Puhl, R. M., C. A. Moss-Racusin, and M. B. Schwartz. 2007. "Internalization of Weight Bias: Implications for Binge Eating and Emotional Well-Being." *Obesity* 15 (1):19–23. doi:10.1038/oby.2007.521.

Rothblum, E. D. 1999. "Contradictions and Confounds in Coverage of Obesity: Psychology Textbooks, Journals, and the Media." *Journal of Social Issues* 55:355–69. doi: 10.1111/0022-4537.00120.

Rothblum, E. D. 2012. "Why a Journal on Fat Studies?" *Fat Studies* 1:3–5. doi: 10.1080/21604851.2012.633469.

Rothblum, E. D., and S. Solovay. 2009. *The Fat Studies Reader*. New York, NY: New York University Press.

Royce, T. 2009. "The Shape of Abuse: Fat Oppression as a Form of Violence against Women." In *The Fat Studies Reader*, Eds. E. Rothblum and S. Solovay, 151–57. New York: New York University Press.

Saguy, A.C. 2013. *What's Wrong With Fat?* New York, NY: Oxford University Press.

Saguy, A.C., and R. Almeling. 2008. "Fat in the Fire? Science, the News Media, and the "Obesity Epidemic." *Sociological Forum* 23:53–83. doi: 10.1111/j.1600-0838.2004.00399.x-i1.

Schafer, M.H., and K.F. Ferraro. 2011. "The Stigma of Obesity: Does Perceived Weight Discrimination Affect Identity and Physical Health?" *Social Psychology Quarterly* 74 (1):76–97. doi:10.1177/0190272511398197.

Schwartz, M. B., L. R. Vartanian, B. A. Nosek, and K. D. Brownell. 2006. "The Influence of One's Own Body Weight on Implicit and Explicit Anti-Fat Bias." *Obesity* 14 (3):440–47. doi:10.1038/oby.2006.58.

Sears, D. O. 1988. "Symbolic Racism." In *Eliminating Racism: Profiles in Controversy*, Eds. P. Katz and D. Taylor, 53–84. New York: Plenum Press.

Sender, K., and M. Sullivan. 2008. "Epidemics of Will, Failures of Self-Esteem: Responding to Fat Bodies in the Biggest Loser and What Not to Wear." *Continuum* 22 (4):573–84. doi:10.1080/10304310802190046.

Skinner, A. C., K. Payne, A. J. Perrin, A. T. Panter, J. B. Howard, A. Bardone-Cone, and E. M. Perrin. 2017. "Implicit Weight Bias in Children Age 9 to 11 Years." *Pediatrics* 140 (1):1–6. doi:10.1542/peds.2016-3936.

Sojka, C. J., and S. Sanchez. 2019. "All People Deserve a Voice in Reproductive Care: Trans-Inclusion in Fat Studies." *Women's Reproductive Health* 6 (4): 259–64.

Sutin, A. R., and A. Terracciano. 2013. "Perceived Weight Discrimination and Obesity." *PloS one* 8 (7):1–8. doi:10.1371/journal.pone.0070048.

Swami, V., L. Steadman, and M. J. Tovée. 2009. "A Comparison of Body Size Ideals, Body Dissatisfaction, and Media Influence between Female Track Athletes, Martial Artists, and Non-Athletes." *Psychology of Sport and Exercise* 10 (6):609–14. doi:10.1016/j.psychsport.2009.03.003.

Sykes, H., and D. McPhail. 2008. "Unbearable Lessons: Contesting Fat Phobia in Physical Education." *Sociology of Sport* 25:66–96. doi: 10.1123/ssj.25.1.66.

Weinstock, J., and M. Krehbiel. 2009. "Fat Youth as Common Targets for Bullying." In *The Fat Studies Reader*, Eds. E. Rothblum and S. Solovay, 120–26. New York: New York University Press.

Whitesel, J. 2017. "Intersections of Multiple Oppressions: Racism, Sizeism, Ableism, and the 'Illimitable Etceteras.' *Sociological Forum* 32(2): 426–33

Wright, J., and V. Harwood. 2009. *Biopolitics and the "Obesity Epidemic": Governing Bodies*. New York, NY: Routledge.

Young, I.M. 1990. "Five Faces of Oppression." In *Justice and the Politics of Difference*, Ed. I.M. Young, 39–63. Princeton, NJ: Princeton University Press.

Crafting weight stigma in slimming classes: A case study in Ireland

Jacqueline O'Toole ⓘ

ABSTRACT

The persistence of dominant social and cultural representations of weight loss renders it as normative and necessary, especially for women. One setting in which the goal of weight loss is relentlessly pursued is the slimming class. Drawn from the analysis of the ethnographic data from a larger one-year narrative inquiry study in four slimming classes in Ireland, this article demonstrates that while slimming is narrated as a positive intervention in the "care of the self," the crafting of weight stigma is central to the dominant weight loss storyline constituted in the classes. Theoretically, the study weaves insights from the feminist expansion of Foucault's work on disciplinary power and governmentality, Goffman's concept of stigma, and narrative inquiry. Three main findings are discussed: the construction of slimming as a quest, slimmer identity, and the overt stigmatizing of fatness. The quest narrative produces a limited set of narrative resources (stories/characters/temporality) that make it very difficult to speak outside the narrative of weight loss. In an Irish context, where the historical circumscription of women's bodies was pervasive, the findings illustrate aspects of the contemporary mechanisms through which such bodily circumscription endures.

Introduction

The pursuit/attainment of a normatively defined body weight has become center staged in most Western societies and requires intense periods of bodywork. Engaging in slimming[1] practices to achieve this is generally a cyclical process, as slimming is overwhelmingly characterized by periods of weight loss, weight maintenance, and weight gain (Monaghan 2008). Commercial slimming classes began to appear in the United Kingdom and the United States in the 1950s. They emerged as popular spaces where people gathered in a public setting to discuss their attempts to lose weight and to seek advice/support and ideas from others. From the beginning they operated as profit-making enterprises (Monaghan, Rich, and Aphramor 2010) and then as now were premised on the idea that sustained weight loss is normative and is best achieved in groups (Allon 1975). The Irish equivalent, Slim Ireland, opened its first classes in Ireland in 1972.[2]

This article is drawn from a wider sociological research study that explored the narrative production of slimming in an Irish context. Adapting Gubrium and Holstein's (2009) threefold conceptual framework of the interplay between narrative frameworks, narrative environments, and narrative practices, I interrogated the links between institutional storytelling and women's personal narratives of slimming in an Irish context. This involved an investigation of how dominant narratives about women and weight management play out in the lives of a group of women immersed in the weekly routines, rhythms, and rituals of a slimming class. Drawing from the ethnographic data, the focus of the current article is on the crafting of weight stigma in the slimming classes and the implications of this for how narratives of weight and body size are constructed and disseminated. Close attention is paid to the organizational embeddedness of narratives, so the voices and preferences of Slim Ireland can be heard (Martin 2002).

Critical perspectives: Challenging "obesity" narratives

As in most Western societies, in Ireland the impetus to lose weight mostly occurs within the moral panic about the "obesity epidemic." However, a wide-ranging body of work has emerged that problematizes and challenges the existence of this alleged "obesity epidemic" (see Boero 2012; Cooper 2016; Monaghan 2008; and in an Irish context, Share and Share 2017). Such research, while theoretically divergent, has critiqued "aspects of the received view on, and responses to, the obesity epidemic" (Clarke 2015, 3). Consequently, it is important to remain wary of the overly simplistic conceptualizations of "obesity" and its alleged outcomes (Lupton 2013) and more useful to interrogate the regimen of "truth" that positions "obesity" as a postmodern epidemic (Boero 2012).

In addition, normative body weight is closely linked to gendered issues of beauty ideals, aesthetics, health, responsible citizenship, moral behavior, and increasing societal and self-surveillance of individual lifestyles (Malson 2008; Tischner 2013). An extensive body of research demonstrates the existence of a set of normative expectations that constitute an ideal body type for women described as the thin, slender, youthful, "fit," and "healthy" body (Bartky 1990; Bordo 2003; Germov and Williams 2008; Mooney, Farley, and Strugnell 2009) and more recently as the thin and toned body (Cairns and Johnson 2015; Gailey 2014). Attaining an ideal body weight enables women to fit into gendered cultural aesthetics *and* demonstrate responsible citizenship through the external presentation of a healthy body and mind (Lupton 1996). The imperative is to achieve a body weight that is *not fat* and *is healthy* with the underpinning assumption that *being fat* and *healthy* are incompatible states of being (Cooper 2016).

It is within this context that I argue that appropriate body size has emerged as a central determinant of social acceptability and social value for women in contemporary Irish society and as a self-evident goal for women (Harjunen 2017). Reliable statistics on women and dieting in Ireland are scant. However, information gleaned from the Health Behaviour in School-Aged Children study in 2010 found that 13.2 percent of children overall reported that they were currently on a diet. This figure has remained stable since 2006. There are statistically significant differences by gender and age group. Overall, 17 percent of girls report trying to lose weight compared to 10 percent of boys, and older children are more likely to report trying to lose weight compared to younger children. There are no statistically significant differences across social class groups. The percentage of children dieting is highest among girls aged 15–17 years old (21.6 percent). Further, as girls got older, they developed increased eating concerns, a higher drive for thinness, and higher levels of body dissatisfaction. The evidence suggests that, like other Western countries, dieting in Ireland begins early in women's lives.

Women in Ireland

Women's bodies have long been a site of contestation in Irish society. Indeed, since the foundation of the Irish State in 1922, the female body has been deeply enmeshed in the intertwining narratives of the nation, family, and religion (Byrne and O'Mahony 2012). Subject to intense surveillance by the Catholic Church and the Irish State, women's sexual and reproductive bodies featured strongly in attempts by the postcolonial Irish nation to carve out a particular Irish identity (Barry 2008; Coulter 1993; Gray and Ryan 1997; O'Connor 2008). Inglis (1998) demonstrates that widespread discourses of regulation and control centering on the reproductive capacities of women's bodies played a key role in defining women's bodies socially and personally. The narrative of the "self-sacrificing Irish mother" demarcated many women's lives. In addition, narratives of control, shame, and guilt framed the field of the corporeal in Irish society, in particularly gendered ways. The female body was considered a site of sin and subject to self-denial and penitential practices (Inglis 2008, 4). The twin goals of modesty and chastity were a requirement for respectable women to display the appearance of being a "good woman" (O'Connor 2005).

There have been profound changes in women's lives in recent decades, and newer narratives of womanhood have emerged. Moreover, the transformation that has occurred in wider Irish society has been largely evidenced and supported by the changes in women's lives from about the 1960s onwards.[3]

Discourses of neoliberalism, individualism, and consumerism are shaping the makeup of Irish society today (Ging 2009). These have been embraced alongside "a realignment of the relationship between Church, state and civil society" (Hill 2003, 5; Inglis 2014). However, the changes that have occurred exhibit uneven trends where gendered social relations and inequalities persist in the face of the "modernization" of Irish society (Connolly 2002; Stokes 2014). What remains, I contend, is a harmful legacy centering on the control of women's bodies. My study addressed ongoing societal concerns with women's bodies through the lens of slimming, an area minimally researched in an Irish context.

Theoretical resources

Engagement in slimming can be theorized as a "body project" that can function as a "practice of the self" proffering the potential of self and corporeal transformation (Reilly et al. 2008). My analysis of how normative meanings of body weight and weight management come to be accepted as "truths" and thereby implicated in the production of narratives of slimming is informed by the feminist expansion of Foucault's work (1977, 1979, 1984, 1988) (see, for example, Heyes 2007; Longhurst 2012; Murray 2008). Accordingly, the tensions between Foucault's repressive and enabling understandings of power and of governmentality highlight the usefulness of his conceptual tool kit. Neoliberal governance extends Foucault's conceptualization of disciplinary power. It operates through techniques of responsibilization that transfer collective responsibility onto individuals who come to self-regulate themselves according to societal requirements and individual choice (Harjunen 2017; Lupton 1996). Widespread structural problems in society are individualized and rendered as private problems that people feel in their everyday lives. Fundamentally, Foucault's analysis illustrates the work involved in modern societies to produce ethically responsible and "normal" citizens whose conduct is shaped by formal political rationalities and by the mundane ways in which individuals govern themselves and others in everyday life (Cairns and Johnson 2015). I consider how the slimming class is a classic exemplar of governmentality *in action*.

Goffman's account of stigma is a second resource drawn on to understand the dynamics of stigma production (Goffman 1963). His theorization of the microlevel experience of stigma as a state of being disqualified from social acceptance is apposite vis-á-vis current debates on fatness and obesity in wider society (Goffman 1963). Sociologically, *stigma* refers to a negatively defined condition, attribute, trait, or behavior conferring "deviant" status that is socially, culturally, and historically variable (Monaghan and Williams 2013). Link and Phelan (2001) extend Goffman's analysis to assert the links between power, structural discrimination, and the responses of stigmatized persons to the labeling that occurs *to* them and *about* them. Tyler (2018) offers a powerful critique of the (over)reliance on Goffman's "apolitical" account of stigma among sociologists. She outlines a conceptual rethinking to examine among other questions: How, why, and by whom stigma is crafted, mediated, and produced (Tyler and Slater 2018, 736).

Data and methods

Slimming is comprised of moral and gendered tales, characterized by multiple stories of "success" and "failure," "before" and "after," and morality tales centering on "good" and "bad" eating patterns and behavior. Positioning slimming as a storied landscape led me to narrative inquiry. It is both a philosophical/theoretical approach that orients the researcher to "storied lives" and a methodological strategy that focuses on the use of stories as data (Elliot 2005; Riessman 2008).[4] Narratives and stories can be strategic, functional, and purposeful (Griffin and May 2012). In this context, Polletta et al. (2011) argue that narratives and stories contribute to the reproduction of existing structures of meaning and power.

I conducted a year-long narrative inquiry study within Slim Ireland.[5] Three methods of data collection were employed in the wider study: non-participant observation in four slimming classes; in-depth, double narrative interviews with 11 women that were digitally recorded and transcribed verbatim; and a narrative analysis of the texts of 32 motivational talks and other Slim Ireland documentation. Once access was achieved, I began attending slimming classes and engaged in nonparticipation observation.[6] For the first few weeks, I introduced myself to each class. At the time of the study, I could be described as being "overweight" and/or "obese" depending on how the BMI calculator was applied. I had also participated in self-directed dieting programs on and off for years. While none of the participants ever questioned me directly about my weight status, the class leaders assumed I was there to lose weight. Indeed, one class leader presented me with a book at one stage that explained how having a large stomach such as mine was caused by holding too much stress in the stomach region. Initially, I took a broad approach to data collection to develop a wide-angle lens view focusing on the general rhythm and routine of each class (Germain 1993). I took brief notes during the classes and wrote these out in detail later. The observations became more focused on listening for stories as the weeks progressed.[7]

I used Lieblich, Tuval-Masiach, and Zilber's (1998) typology of narrative analysis, which consists of a matrix of four cells, consisting of four modes of reading a narrative: *holistic form, holistic content, categorical form, and categorical content*. I deployed a holistic-form approach to analyze the field notes and documents from Slim Ireland. Initially, I conducted a detailed examination of the observation field notes, postobservation write-ups, and the texts of the motivational talks to develop what Lieblich, Tuval-Masiach, and Zilber (1998) term a "global impression." This enabled a sketch of the progression of the plot. Multiple readings of the field notes led to a visualization of the emerging story. A two-stage analysis was deployed. First, a thematic focus for the development of the plot was identified (Lieblich, Tuval-Masiach, and Zilber 1998, 89; O' Toole 2018). Content is important here to provide raw material for the structure. The second stage characterized the dynamics of the plot inferred from particular forms of speech (Lieblich, Tuval-Masiach, and Zilber 1998, 91). I focused on the use of recurring specific phrases and the use of terms that expressed the structural component of the narrative.[8]

Findings

The quest narrative: Slimming for a "better" body

The weekly classes provided a regular form of monitoring and support in the pursuit of weight loss. When a woman joins such a class, she ostensibly "signs up" to this monitoring. Slim Ireland attempts to establish order, structure, and routine around food and eating patterns, exercise, and general "well-being" in the lives of its members. The holistic-form analysis of the ethnographic data revealed that the stories told within the slimming class drew from what Frank (1995) conceptualizes as the quest narrative, and this dominates the practice of storytelling in the slimming classes.

All quests begin with a call, represented in this study as "turning points." These include wanting to fit into clothes, attending significant life events, body dis-satisfaction/hatred, and ill health. The specifics of the quest template constituted by Slim Ireland emphasized biographical interruption due to perceived suffering (becoming "overweight"), facing up to the challenge/overcoming obstacles (subjecting oneself to the regimen of weight loss), and ultimately, achieving self-transformation. This is illustrated in the following excerpt from field notes:

> You are lacking in self-control and eat too much. We share that problem and can help you. Our philosophy is based on years of experience of helping loads of people just like you. I have been there but now I'm better. Stick with us and you will succeed. (Field work notes, Class 3)

This version of the weight loss narrative is told and retold every week in the slimming class to both emphasize its importance *and* to generate a coherent weight loss story to pursue a "better" body. In so doing, the slimming class facilitates what Martin (2002) enunciates as frame alignment with organizational identity. What this also illustrates is that in signing up to a class, from the outset the woman's body is constructed as discredited in Goffman's terms.

The idea of slimming as a necessary and ethical body project underpins the quest narrative and is constituted as having a linear progressive temporality, moving over time, from "overweight" and/or "obese" to "normal" weight. It is also paradoxically positioned as potentially lifelong and full of struggle. There is always a chance that women will fail at weight loss, and the class leaders constantly reminded women of this: "The weeks leading up to Christmas can be more dangerous than Christmas itself" (Bernie, Class 3 leader during one of her speaking segments).

To enforce its message, Slim Ireland only tells certain stories in the classes that ultimately serve to reduce weight loss to a simplistic set of behaviors: "It's really so simple, once the light switches on, it stays on. And *then* you lose weight" (Field work notes, Class 4).

The whole class is then built around conveying this message of "mind over matter," an exemplar of the mind/body dualism that permeates much discussion on weight loss.

The women are also constrained in the kinds of stories they can tell. Usually, these are confessional stories that tend to be underpinned by stories of being out of control, of having insatiable appetites, of denouncing fatness, and of seeking ways to overcome the challenges these present.

For example:

> Another woman who weighs in is told by Bernie to have a clean slate next week as she has put loads of weight on. This woman has found it difficult to lose weight and tells Bernie that she has a lot going on in her life. Bernie sighs and says "So be it. We all have a lot going on but what do we want from this class, to get bigger? I don't think so." The woman tries to explain that she mostly sticks to the plans, but it is hard to be "good all the time." Bernie tells her to at least "be good some of the time." The woman returns to her seat but seems despondent. She tells other women around her that she has been going through a lot with work and the children and how hard it is to lose the weight. They all nod to signal quiet agreement. (Field work notes, Class 3)

Demands are placed on members to recount to others their personal transgressions of excess and indulgence. Some stories are more tellable than others in this context. *Failure to lose weight* stories can be publicly told in the slimming class but are generally told within a frame of accountability, as these two excerpts from the field notes indicate:

> For most of the women bread seems to be one food that is discussed often. Women think of bread as both enemy and friend, but it seems mainly enemy. Many conversations with Maggie [leader] begin with stories of bread: how much bread is eaten, how often it is eaten, what types of bread are eaten. There is a sense that they are confessing each week about bread, sometimes potatoes and other foods, but if I heard it once, I heard it many times: "Bread is my downfall." (Field work notes, Class 1)

> I hear snippets of other stories that begin and then trail off: "I know I'm not taking this too seriously as I only do a little bit of what she tells us"; "God, I had such a stressful week with the kids and everything. I never got a minute to myself to prepare and work at this." (Field work notes, Class 3)

Accounting for self is central to both weight-loss narratives and to gender narratives. This is followed closely by attempts to seek atonement. Mycroft (2008) states that morality and accountability permeate slimming classes and are grounded in the judgment of women. The mechanics of accountability are borne out in the hegemonic character at the heart of the quest: the "successful slimmer."

Slimmer identity

To support the quest narrative, Slim Ireland worked hard to mobilize a coherent slimmer identity for its members through its promotional materials, practices, and motivational talks within the classes. This was illustrated on many occasions through a story about what makes a "bad" slimmer. Frank (1995) points out that moral work takes place in storytelling. For example, class leaders offered explanations as to why many women appear to have no control when it comes to food and eating practices. The nebulous concepts of "emotional hunger" and "emotional appetites" are center-staged:

> Eating only sorts out, cures hunger, nothing else. When did you last crave a bowl of porridge, carrots, cabbage? How do I know when it [hunger] is real? When it's just a craving? We need to take a step back, take twenty minutes and drink water, and then if we still feel hungry we can eat. Emotional hunger is uncontrollable. We say we can't stop ourselves, but we can. We need to blame ourselves... . This started early in life by reaching for something. The biggest thing is to take responsibility. You and only you takes [sic] the food. No one else puts the food into your mouth. Take responsibility and ask yourself why you are overeating. Write it down. I see it on the scales you know [much laughter in the room]! Look, I've seen members put their hands over a scone in a shop. I'm not eating it, you are. If you should eat it then you wouldn't be hiding. (Field work notes Class 3)

The insatiable nature of women's appetites is invoked here, as is the problematic category of blame. There is an attempt to limit understandings of "overeating" to an emotionally fraught self in need of attention. Members are continually asked to reflect on why they "eat so much" and why they feel the need to eat so regularly. The role of the narrator is important here. She tends to use "we" and "I" to signal identification with the Slim Ireland narrative. The leader mixes the written text provided by Slim Ireland with her own anecdotes to convey the message that engaging in out-of-control eating is firmly located in emotional desires and cravings that can and must be defeated.

The exemplar of the slimmer identity is the "successful slimmer" who is held up to all who attend the classes as a counter to the "out-of-control" character. A hegemonic character, she makes an appearance in the promotional literature but also during the "celebration" of the weight-loss segment that takes place during every class. Here, the woman who successfully loses the most weight each week is given special mention in the class—where her "success story" has the potential to be everyone's "success story" if the quest is followed correctly. Her story is the benchmark for both success and failure. As Herndon (2008) observes, the paradox remains that while dieting has become normalized, those who have lost weight continue to be put on pedestals and their efforts admired. To commit to becoming a "successful slimmer" holds the reward of acquiring a "less" stigmatized, morally presentable self, made visible through the slim(mer) body:

> Slim people are slim because they take RESPONSIBILITY for what they eat and how they live. They don't need to be told what to do all the time. They decide for themselves how to eat and exercise. You will become slim once you decide to take responsibility for your decisions.... Successful people are also totally FOCUSED... . Successful people also take CONTROL.... You have the power to control your weight, not the other way around. By taking more control of your eating, you take more control of your life. (Motivational talk 36/08)

Nonslim people are depicted as irresponsible, unfocused, and out of control. But they are also encouraged to learn from the habits of "normal" (code = slim) people.

Overt stigmatizing of fatness

The quest is heightened by the refusal to acknowledge that fatness might be anything other than a "spoiled" identity and stigmatized status for women. According to Slim Ireland, a better body is a less fat body and preferably a nonfat body. There were many overt expressions of fat phobia within the classes. In one class a poster placed at the sign-in /merchandise table displayed the tagline "A Flabby Body Is a Flabby Mind." In another class, the class leader brought in a lump of lard weighing about 3 kilograms (6.6 pounds) packaged in a clear plastic bag. She placed it on the table for all to comment. She explained to everyone that this is what fat looks like and how disgusting it was to be carrying this around on one's body every day. Lupton (2014) describes how the "pedagogy of disgust" that permeates many public health campaigns around diet and exercise has normative effects. Thus, deploying disgust has the effect of continually emphasizing the dangers of internal and external fatness. This was reinforced in another class when I mentioned HAES® to the class leader. As a thin woman who was, in her own words "constantly watching her weight," she was incredulous and stated quite categorically that "No one could ever think it is okay to be fat. No one is ever happy to be fat. No one."

Bernie (class leader, Class 3) referenced fat/fatness pejoratively through a rehearsed story that she told at different intervals during my time observing in Class 3:

> Bernie is delivering the motivational talk. The theme this week is "Change not chance will get you to this. Life is not a dress rehearsal." Bernie mentions Úna,

who has lost a half a stone (7 pounds) in two weeks. She tells everyone that Úna is not more special than anyone else. Úna just works hard. She asks us are we living life to the full and somebody says no! "Well," says Bernie, "weight does that, it does slow us down and leaves us open to different kinds of infections. You want to change, don't you?" We all nod in the affirmative. "It will happen," Bernie tells us. "You must put everything into place. One pound a week and you will all have a stone off by Easter. One pound a week for the year and that is 4 stone, folks. Losing weight will change your life, your energy. Look let me. Let me tell you all something. I've been there, yes, I have. I know it all. You see, I've lost five and a half stone. I was always fat: a fat baby, a fat child, a fat teenager, a fat adult. By the time I was 14, I was 14 stone. But I didn't have happy teenage years. Once in class, a nun called me a "baby elephant." We all exclaim. Bernie continues. "I know what it's like. I don't have a halo. I face the same battles as you do. Oh yeah, I put on four pounds over Christmas and now I've shifted two but these other two are staying for now. I know it's there. It's as hard for me as for you." (Field work notes, Class 3)

Within this encounter Bernie locates herself as an ally of the members in their weight-loss efforts. She reinforces this identification with the constant use of "I." Drawing on the narrative device of identification, Bernie is telling the members that she too has experienced the perceived problems associated with being fat: "It's as hard for me as for you." This enables all in the room to identify as having similar experiences, which is a useful tool in an organization's attempts to inscribe its narrative on its members.

Discussion

Narrative inquiry is a useful approach to excavate institutional storytelling, to illustrate how temporal unity is maintained through the use of a plot, and to attend to the normalizing power of dominant narratives. The normative function of narrative environments is to craft a persuasive and meaningful story for the audience, to sediment a coherent narrative (Andersen 2015). In this regard, the slimming class is one key narrative environment. Slim Ireland constructs slimming as a quest for a "better" body, ultimately casting the quest as a positive intervention in the "care of the self" (Gill, Henwood, and McLean 2005). It draws from neoliberal narratives to situate normative body weight as fundamental to responsible and moral citizenship. Further, by adopting an orthodox position on the "obesity as epidemic" narrative that links weight loss to health, normative femininity, and improved quality of life, it promotes its role to transform and reform recalcitrant bodies and selves. The demands for constant micromanagement and surveillance also illustrate the operation of the normalizing bodily practices of biopower in everyday life (Tischner 2013). Slim Ireland requires self-government while simultaneously translating expert discourses on diet and "obesity" into concrete techniques for governing the dieting self (Clarke 2015).

The increasing importance of the "biographical project of the self" carries with it a powerful (and new) form of governance (Rose 1999). The authentic and fully realized self is subject to continual (self-) surveillance, transformation, and improvement, in a process that has long formed a central element of normative femininity. In the neoliberal social order, there is an imperative on individual subjects to construct and display themselves as distinctive, authentic selves; discerning consumers; and as ethical subjects. If one behaves in ways that are taken to be excessive, unhealthy, irresponsible, or undisciplined, then this is constituted as a moral failure of the self. Neoliberal ideals of self-control and exhibiting control in all facets of one's life, including eating, exercising, and having a socially defined body weight, are enmeshed in weight management narratives (Cairns and Johnson 2015).

What is concealed in the quest narrative, however, is that which underpins the quest *itself*—a crafting of weight stigma in ways that serve to embed fat phobia at micro (individual), meso (slimming practices), and macro (policy, media etc.) levels. Throsby (2009, 201–202) describes how the failure to lose weight is seen as "evidence of a moral failure of individual responsibility to care appropriately for the self, and by extension, to be a good citizen." Society effectively sanctions fatness as failure. In this sense, the crafting of weight stigma in the slimming classes echoes Scambler's (2018) conceptualization of the "weaponizing" of stigma in the neoliberal era. For Scambler (2018) the key to understanding stigma production in contemporary societies lies more specifically in the capitalist social structure and class relations in society. This clearly goes "beyond Goffman" but does not completely negate him, as Scambler (2018, 768) himself attests: "What is missing [in Goffman] … is the casual role of social structures, like class, command, gender, ethnicity, and so on." In my study, the focus was on gender and weight structures. In narrating slimming as a quest, the slimming class constructs fatness as an offense against norms of shame (normative body size) and norms of gender (the "good" woman).

Previously in Ireland, women's "good citizenship" was closely monitored in the "private" and "domestic" space, evident in a century of laws prohibiting the choice to work and in the regulation of fertility, for example. Arguably, women's "private" lives were in fact "public" property, whereby the "good" of the nation was located in the regulation of women's everyday lives. Evidently, the narrative nexus surrounding women's lives, once dominated by Catholicism and the State and centered on women's bodies and the family, has shifted in recent decades. Notwithstanding, I contend that women in Ireland continue to have to account for themselves in particularly gendered ways. Moreover, much of this is drawn from contemporary moral concerns about women's bodies—what they look like and how much they weigh. Corporeal experiences such as those enmeshed in slimming continue to be implicated in the construction of the "good woman" in Irish society.

Notes

1. In Ireland, the term *slimming* is the general term used to refer to an array of weight management practices that elsewhere are described as dieting and/or weight loss. Included are food monitoring and restriction, exercise, attending weight management classes, following online weight loss programs, and so forth. I use the terms *slimming* and *dieting* interchangeably in this article.

2. Slim Ireland is a pseudonym. *Ireland* refers to the whole island of Ireland and comprises the Republic of Ireland and Northern Ireland. My study took place in the Republic of Ireland. Northern Ireland is part of the United Kingdom. Slim Ireland operates in both jurisdictions.

3. Positive changes include increased participation in the paid labor force; equal pay; the introduction of divorce; proposed new legislation to guarantee reproductive rights, including abortion; the criminalization of rape both within and outside marriage; marriage equality for LGTBT people; and so forth.

4. I use the terms *story* and *narrative* interchangeably.

5. Full ethical approval was received from the Research Ethics Committee in the National University of Ireland, Galway, prior to contacting any commercial weight loss organization. Slim Ireland received all the necessary participation information and consent documentation and was fully apprised of the nature of the research process before and during the observation period.

6. Negotiating and gaining access to the organization is discussed in more detail elsewhere (O' Toole 2018).

7. The process of sampling and recruiting women to interview began in the first class. A multistage purposeful sampling process generated a final sample of 11 women, 9 women members and 2 class leaders. The women identified as White and Irish, were from rural backgrounds, ranged in age from 27–67, and had been engaged in slimming practices for many years. Each woman was interviewed twice: The first interview "schedule" was an adapted Biographical Narrative Inquiry Method (Wengraf 2001), which involved asking only one question at the beginning and then letting the interview flow. The second interview was a semistructured interview using an interview schedule devised from a preliminary thematic analysis of interview one and other key issues I wished to explore.

8. The interview texts were subjected to both a holistic-form analysis, following similar procedures as with the field notes/documentation, and a categorical-content analysis to analyze both the *whats* and the *hows* of storytelling. The latter proceeds similar to thematic analysis. What differentiates it is that the selected data are not fractured nor isolated from the personal contexts from which they emanated.

ORCID

Jacqueline O'Toole ⓘ http://orcid.org/0000-0003-0362-8744

References

Allon, N. 1975. "Latent Social Services in Group Dieting." *Social Problems* 23 (1):56–59. doi:10.2307/799628

Andersen, D. 2015. "Stories of Change in Drug Treatment: A Narrative Analysis of "Whats" and "Hows" in Institutional Storytelling." *Sociology of Health & Illness* 37 (5):668–82. doi:10.1111/1467-9566.12228

Barry, U. 2008. *Where are We Now: New Feminist Perspectives on Women in Contemporary Ireland*. Dublin: TASC New Ireland.

Bartky, S.L. 1990. *Femininity and Domination: Studies in the Phenomenology of Oppression*. New York: Routledge.

Boero, N. 2012. *Killer Fat: Media, Medicine and Morals in the American "Obesity Epidemic"*. New Brunswick, NJ: Rutgers University Press.

Bordo, S. 2003. *Unbearable Weight: 10th Anniversary Edition*. Berkeley: University of California.

Byrne, A., and D. O'Mahony. 2012. "Family and Community: (Re)Telling Our Own Story." *Journal of Family Issues* 33 (1):52–75. doi:10.1177/0192513X11421121

Cairns, K., and J. Johnson. 2015. "Choosing Health: Embodied Neoliberalism, Postfeminism, and the "Do-Diet" *Theory and Society* 44 (2):153–75. doi:10.1007/s11186-015-9242-y

Clarke, A.C. 2015. "Governing the Dieting Self: Conducting Weight –Loss via the Internet." *Journal of Sociology* 15 (51):657–73. doi:10.1177/1440783314522869

Connolly, L. 2002. *The Irish Women's Movement*. New York: Palgrave.

Cooper, C. 2016. *Fat Activism: A Radical Social Movement*. Bristol: HammerOn Press.

Coulter, C. 1993. *The Hidden Tradition: Feminism, Women and Nationalism in Ireland*. Cork: Mercier Press.

Elliot, J. 2005. *Using Narrative in Social Research: Qualitative and Quantitative Approaches*. London: SAGE.

Foucault, M. 1977. *Discipline and Punish: The Birth of the Prison*. London: Penguin.

Foucault, M. 1979. *The History of Sexuality, Volume 1: An Introduction*. Harmondsworth: Penguin.

Foucault, M. 1984. *The History of Sexuality Volume 2: The Uses of Pleasure*. London: Penguin.

Foucault, M. 1988. "Technologies of the Self." In *Technologies of the Self*, edited by L. Martin, H. Gutman, and P. H. Hutton, 16–49. London: Tavistoock.

Frank, A.W. 1995. *The Wounded Storyteller: Body, Illness and Ethics*. Chicago: University of Chicago Press.

Gailey, J. 2014. *The hyper(In)visible Fat Woman*. New York: Palgrave Macmillan.

Germain, C. 1993. "Ethnography: The Method." In *Nursing Research: A Qualitative Perspective*, edited by P. Munhall and C. Oiler Boyd, 147–162, 2nd ed. New York, NY: National League for Nursing.

Germov, J., and L. Williams. 2008. *A Sociology of Food and Nutrition: The Social Appetite*. Australia: Oxford University Press.

Gill, R., K. Henwood, and C. McLean. 2005. "Body Projects and the Regulation of Normative Masculinity." *Body & Society* 11 (1):37–62. doi:10.1177/1357034X05049849

Ging, D. 2009. "All-Consuming Images: New Gender Formations in post-Celtic-tiger Ireland." In *Transforming Ireland: Challenges, Critiques and Resources*, edited by D. Ging, M. Cronin, and P. Kirby, 52–70. Manchester: Manchester University Press.

Goffman, E. 1963. *Stigma: Notes on the Management of Spoiled Identity*. New York: Simon and Schuster.

Gray, B., and L. Ryan. 1997. "(Dis)Locating "Woman" and Women in Representations of Irish Nationality." In *Women in Irish Society*, edited by A. Byrne and M. Leonard, 517–534. Belfast: Beyond the Pale Publications.

Griffin, A., and V. May. 2012. "Narrative Analysis and Interpretative Phenomenological Analysis." In *Researching Society and Culture*, edited by C. Seale, 441–458, 3rd ed. London: Sage.

Gubrium, J.F., and J. A. Holstein. 2009. *Analysing Narrative Reality*. Thousand Oaks, CA: Sage.

Harjunen, H. 2017. *Neoliberal Bodies and the Gendered Fat Body*. London: Routledge.

Herndon, A. M. 2008. "Taking the Devil into Your Mouth: Ritualised American Weight Loss Narratives of Morality, Pain and Betrayal." *Perspectives in Biology and Medicine* 51 (2):207–19. doi:10.1353/pbm.0.0004

Heyes, C.J. 2007. *Self-Transformations: Foucault, Ethics, and Normalised Bodies*. New York: Oxford University Press.

Hill, M. 2003. *Women in Ireland: A Century of Change*. Belfast: Blackstaff Press.

Inglis, T. 1998. *Moral Monopoly: The Rise and Fall of the Catholic Church in Modern Ireland*. Dublin: UCD Press.

Inglis, T. 2008. *Global Ireland: Same Difference*. New York: Routledge.

Inglis, T. 2014. *Are the Irish Different?* Manchester: Manchester University Press.

Lieblich, A., R. Tuval-Masiach, and T. Zilber. 1998. *Narrative Research: Reading, Analysis and Interpretation*. Thousand Oaks CA: Sage.

Link, B. G., and J. C. Phelan. 2001. "Conceptualizing Stigma." *Annual Review of Sociology* 27: 363–85. doi: 10.1146/annurev.soc.27.1.363.

Longhurst, R. 2012. "Becoming Smaller: Autobiographical Spaces of Weight Loss." *Antipode* 44: 871–88. doi: 10.1111/j.1467-8330.2011.00895.x.

Lupton, D. 1996. *Food, the Body and the Self*. London: Sage.

Lupton, D. 2013. *Fat*. London: Routledge.

Lupton, D. 2014. "The Pedagogy of Disgust: The Ethical, Moral and Political Implications of Using Disgust in Public Health Campaigns." *Critical Public Health* 25 (1):1–11.

Malson, H. 2008. "Deconstructing Un/Healthy Body-Weight and Weight Management." In *Critical Bodies: Representations, Identities and Practices of Weight and Body Management*, edited by S. Reilly, M. Burns, H. Frith, S. Wiggins, and P. Markula, 27–42. Basingstoke: Palgrave Macmillan.

Martin, D. 2002. "From Appearance Tales to Oppression Tales: Frame Alignment and Organisational Identify." *Journal of Contemporary Ethnography* 31 (2):158–206. doi:10.1177/0891241602031002003

Monaghan, L. 2008. *Men and the War on Obesity*. London: Routledge.

Monaghan, L., E. Rich, and L. Aphramor. 2010. "Reflections on and Developing Critical Weight Studies." In *Debating Obesity: Critical Perspectives*, edited by E. Rich, L. Monaghan, and L. Aphramor, 219–258. London: Palgrave Macmillan.

Monaghan, L., and S. Williams. 2013. "Stigma." In *Key Concepts in Medical Sociology*, edited by J. Gabe and L. Monaghan, 58–62, 2nd ed. London: Sage.

Mooney, E., H. Farley, and C. Strugnell. 2009. "A Qualitative Investigation into the Opinions of Adolescent Females regarding Their Body Image Concerns and Dieting Practices in the Republic of Ireland." *Appetite* 52: 485–91. doi: 10.1016/j.appet.2008.12.012.

Murray, S. 2008. *The "Fat" Female Body*. New York, NY: Palgrave Macmillan.

Mycroft, H. 2008. "Morality and Accountability in a Commercial Weight Management Group." *Journal of Health Psychology* 13 (8):1040–50. doi:10.1177/1359105308097969

O' Toole, J. 2018. "Institutional Storytelling and Personal Narratives: Reflecting on the 'Value' of Narrative Inquiry' in O'Grady, G., J. O'Toole and D.J. Clandinin, Journal of the Educational Studies Association of Ireland Special Issue: Engaging in Narrative Inquiry." London: Routledge/Taylor & Francis Group. *Making Visible Alternative Knowledge* 37 (2):175–89.

O'Connor, B. 2005. "Sexing the Nation: Discourses of the Dancing Body in Ireland in the 1930s." *Journal of Gender Studies* 14 (2):89–105. doi:10.1080/09589230500133502

O'Connor, P. 2008. "The Irish Patriarchal State: Continuity and Change." In *Contesting the State: Lessons from the Irish Case*, edited by M. Adshead, P. Kirby, and M. Millar, 146–164. Manchester: Manchester University Press.

Polletta, F., B.C Pang Ching, B. Gharrity Gardner, and A. Motes. 2011. "The Sociology of Storytelling." *Annual Review Sociology* 37: 109–30. doi: 10.1146/annurev-soc-081309-150106.

Reilly, S., M. Burns, H. Frith, S. Wiggins, and P. Markula. 2008. *Critical Bodies: Representations, Identities and Practices of Weight and Body Management*. Basingstoke: Palgrave Macmillan.

Riessman, C.K. 2008. *Narrative Methods for the Human Sciences*. London: Sage.

Rose, N. 1999. *Governing the Soul: The Shaping of the Private Self*. 2nd ed. London: Free Association Books.

Scambler, G. 2018. "Heaping Blame on Shame: "Weaponising Stigma" for Neoliberal Times." *The Sociological Review Monographs* 66 (4):766–82. doi:10.1177/0038026118778177

Share, M., and P. Share. 2017. "Doing the "Right Thing"? Children, Families and Fatness in Ireland." In *Reframing Health and Health Policy in Ireland: A Governmental Analysis*, edited by C. Edwards and E. Fernandez, 46–71. Manchester: Manchester University Press.

Stokes, S. 2014. "The Cheap Lock and the Master Key: Raunch Culture's Double Standard and Its Impact on Irish Women's Sexual Lives." In *Sexualities and Irish Society: A Reader*, edited by M. Leane and E. Kiely, 401–418. London: Orpen Press.

Throsby, K. 2009. "The War on Obesity as a Moral Project: Weight Loss Drugs, Obesity Surgery and Negotiating Failure." *Science as Culture* 18 (1):201–16. doi:10.1080/09505430902885581

Tischner, I. 2013. *Fat Lives: A Feminist Psychological Exploration*. New York, NY: Routledge.

Tyler, I. 2018. "Resituating Erving Goffman: From Stigma to Black Power." *The Sociological Review Monographs* 66 (4):744–65. doi:10.1177/0038026118777450

Tyler, I., and T. Slater. 2018. "Rethinking the Sociology of Stigma." *The Sociological Review Monographs* 66 (4):721–43. doi:10.1177/0038026118777425

Wengraf, T. 2001. *Qualitative Research Interviewing: Biographic Narrative and Semi-Structured Methods*. London: Sage.

Understanding fatness: Jamaican women's constructions of health

Claudia Barned and Kieran O'Doherty

ABSTRACT

The prevalence of dominant health discourses has been observed in many Western countries. These discourses tend to associate fatness with ill health, perpetuating stigma and negative attributions about bigger bodies. The authors examine women's constructions of health in an urban Jamaican context. The findings show that women generally reproduce the dominant (Western) "obesity epidemic" discourse, but also take up a local cultural discourse, which the authors call the slim-thick healthy body discourse. The authors describe the features of this discourse and contrast it with the dominant "obesity epidemic" discourse. They conclude by considering both positive and negative implications of both discourses and suggest possibilities for challenging them.

Introduction

In the West, fatness is generally framed as a social problem or a medical liability in need of urgent attention (Gard and Wright 2005; Kwan and Graves 2013). Interpreting fatness in this manner perpetuates stigma and negative attributions about bigger bodies. Talk about fatness largely depends on social factors, such as culture, race, and gender (Abou-Rizk and Rail 2014). Much of what is known about the dominant construction of fatness is situated within a Western purview, with very few studies examining the discursive constructions of ethnic minority groups or people living in non-North American contexts (see Abou-Rizk and Rail 2014; George and Rail 2006; Rice 2014).

The purpose of this study w to examine Jamaican women's understanding of health in relation to dominant global and local health discourses. Despite studies on body image, health, and standards of beauty in Jamaica (Barned and Lipps 2014; Mohammed 2000; Pearce, Dibb, and Gaines 2014; Sobo 1993; Tate 2007), little is known about the discourses that are available in this cultural setting, and the effects they may have on women's health and bodily practices. The present study was a component of the first author's doctoral research, which explored notions of health and beauty in urban Jamaica. Participants were interviewed about their conceptualizations of health and beauty and related bodily practices. In the sections that follow, we review the body image literature on Black resistance to Euro-American understandings of health and beauty.

Hegemonically defined beauty norms and Black resistance

Scholars have argued that from the times of slavery and colonialism, Black beauty has been placed as other compared to Whiteness (Tate 2007, 2013). The Euro-American standard of beauty that is characterized by a White, thin, and toned body has been described as both stringent and marginalizing (Jafar and Casanova 2013; Patton 2006), particularly for those with intersecting marginalized identities, such as being female, fat, and Black. Such bodies reportedly deviate too far from the White/thin ideal and are often labeled as grotesque, abject, and unfeminine (Hobson 2003; Rice 2014). Women from racialized backgrounds navigate a world where their bodies are judged harshly based on the color of their skin, the size of their body, nose and lips, and the texture of their hair as well as its length (Tate 2007, 2013). Studies suggest that racialized women negotiate these constraints by sub-scribing to a beauty culture that is more inclusive of their own norms and values (Barned 2017; Gentles-Peart 2013; Tull et al. 2001; Wilk 1995).

Most studies exploring standards of beauty in African or Caribbean con-texts (e.g. Gentles-Peart 2013; Tull et al. 2001; Wilk 1995) have found that the participants often subscribe to beauty cultures that are very different from Eurocentric ideals. For example, Gentles-Peart (2013) found that the Caribbean participants in her study all subscribed to a beauty culture that endorsed fatness, in particular, a voluptuous, curvaceous figure. The partici-pants in her study spoke extensively about the difference in beauty standards between the Caribbean/West Indies and the United States. One participant in particular suggested that perhaps it is a "West Indian thing" (Gentles-Peart 2013, 32) to find larger, thicker girls more attractive.

In addition to the cultural component, Gentles-Peart (2013) noted that in particular contexts there may also be racial attributions. Research exploring such issues has found that among Caribbean nationals, the dominant Western beauty ideal is referred to as the White shape (thin with no curves), while the thick, Coca-Cola bottle and curvaceous figure is referred to as the Black shape (Anderson-Fye 2004; Gentles-Peart 2013). These studies suggest that for Caribbean nationals, beauty is intricately related to race and racial identity.

Researchers who have found that Black women subscribe to White ideals have also noted that they do so with slight resistance (Miller 1969; Patton

2006). Patton argued that over several years Africans and African Americans have used many resistance strategies to challenge hegemonically-defined beauty norms in the United States. The counterhegemonic creation of unique hairstyles such as dreadlocks and plaits, as well as hair accessories such as scarves, headbands, and weaves, showcased Black beauty and creativity, and worked well as acts of resistance toward Eurocentric ideals of beauty (Patton 2006; Tate 2013). Patton noted that such popular resistant strategies were most visible during the Black Power movement that simultaneously promoted the "Black is Beautiful" campaign. This campaign led to the creation of a counter discourse that opposes mainstream Eurocentric beauty standards promoting Whiteness. The Black Power movement, through the use of the "Black is Beautiful" campaign, worked toward altering the racist stereotypes that insisted that Black was ugly and undesirable (Patton 2006).

The Black Power movement in the United States challenged the ingrained stereotypes of beauty that were and are still perpetuated by Euro-Americans. Patton (2006) argued that African American women need to continue challenging the notion of White hegemonic beauty as the norm and to demand the recognition of diversified Black beauty. According to Patton, it is only through acknowledging and recognizing that other forms of beauty exist beyond Euro-American definitions, that one is able to understand that there are different types of beauty in the world. Patton argues that it is because of this counter discourse that there is a wider range of beauty norms and acceptance of a variety of body types and sizes among people of African descent.

In contemporary Jamaican society, resistance to the Eurocentric ideal is evident through the emergence and island-wide uptake of the term *fluffy* (Pearce, Dibb, and Gaines 2014). The term was coined by Jamaican emcee Khadine Hylton (commonly known as "Miss Kitty"), and has become a popular adjective used to describe plump or big-bodied women who are confident in their appearance. The term is gender and age specific, and generally only young to middle-aged women are referred to as fluffy (Barned and Lipps 2014). While the term is used globally to describe inanimate objects or animals, it has gained a new meaning in Jamaican society when it became associated with big-bodied women who medically would be considered "overweight." This unique interpretation of fatness suggests that in the Jamaican cultural context, fatness is not only endorsed, but is also culturally valued. Pearce, Dibb, and Gaines referred to this valuing as a form of disidentifying with the colonial or European notion of thin as ideal, and a rebranding of fluffy as the Afro-Caribbean ideal.

Interpretations of fatness in Jamaica

The aforementioned studies suggest that in Jamaica, the meanings ascribed to big bodies extend beyond associating size with eating patterns and dietary habits; they also include inferences about health and beauty. For example, Sobo (1993) reported that thin bodies in rural Jamaica were seen as weak, infertile, and antisocial, whereas fat bodies were linked with kindness, fertility, vitality, and bodily health. Savacool (2009) reported similar findings, whereby voluptuous, plump, or full-figured women were described more favorably and considered more attractive than thin women. Pearce, Dibb, and Gaines (2014) and Barned (2017) found that Jamaicans typically describe a healthy body as one that is "not too fat," "not too skinny," "medium," "plump" or "thick." Unlike the dominant meanings ascribed to fat bodies in North America and Europe, these findings suggest that within Jamaican society, fatness is indicative of both health and beauty.

Fat studies approach

In this study, we take a critical feminist lens to explore how bodies are read and positioned in urban Jamaica. To do this, we first discuss the implications of a dominant health discourse documented in the literature, that is, "obesity" discourse (Rail and Lafrance 2009; Rich and Evans 2005), otherwise called "obesity" epidemic discourse (Gard and Kirk 2007). Researchers have written about this discourse from a critical perspective (see Lawrence 2004; Rail 2012; Rich and Evans 2005), often adopting a critical stance to "obesity" science research and representations of fatness as "obesity."

Critical health researchers have argued that this discourse labels fat bodies as at-risk, lazy, abject, and problematic (Rail and Lafrance 2009; Rice 2014), based on the notion that thin bodies represent the "gold standard of health." Bodies that fall outside of the thin category are typically considered abnormal or deviant. Uptake of this discourse is characterized by an endorsement of thinness, as well as the overall promotion of weight control as an unquestionable health practice. According to Rail (2012), key features of this discourse include interpreting "obesity": (a) as a disease, (b) as being directly related to health problems, (c) as an outcome of lifestyle choices, (d) as a personal responsibility, and (e) as a global epidemic. Other features include: (f) interpreting claims about "obesity" as facts based on biomedical reports and expert opinions and (g) interpreting weight loss as the solution for "obesity" and improved health (230–239).

Several studies have focused on constructions of health within the context of the "obesity" epidemic discourse (Abou-Rizk and Rail 2014; Rail 2010; Rail, Holmes, and Murray 2010; Wright, O'Flynn, and Macdonald 2006). A common finding is that women consistently highlight the importance of physical activity, a balanced diet, and maintaining an appropriate weight (Abou-Rizk and Rail 2012; George and Rail 2006). For example, the South Asian women in George and Rail's (2006) study and the Lebanese Canadian women in Abou-Rizk and Rail's (2014) study all constructed health using elements of the "obesity" epidemic discourse, whereby they likened health with looking good and not being fat. The authors found that women's constructions of health were all situated in discussions about "obesity" and weight; the young women in their study reproduced aspects of the "obesity" epidemic discourse, that is, negative messages that perpetuate discriminatory information about fat bodies.

Lebanese Canadian women reported that their idea of a healthy body was similar to that of an average-sized body, one that would be characterized as "normal," that is, not too fat and not too thin (Abou-Rizk and Rail 2014). However, when situating this body on a continuum, it was described as being closer to thin than to fat. The majority of the women in their study expressed a desire for a thin or skinny body; however, some noted that there is not one perfect body size or shape that represents health and beauty. They showed "significant levels of awareness of the dominant discourses that dictate how they should look to be considered 'healthy' and 'beautiful'," yet also seemed to be "caught in a vicious cycle of abidance to the societal norms and rules perpetuated by these discourses" (9). Abou-Rizk and Rail further found that while almost all of their participants expressed some form of negativity toward "overweight" or "obese" bodies, some of them also ridiculed the thin body, and discussed its inappropriateness as a cultural beauty ideal. They argued that such a cultural ideal is unattainable, unrealistic, and at times, even unhealthy. These participants engaged in what Abou-Rizk and Rail referred to as light resistance to the dominant discourses of conventional femininity and "obesity."

These studies emphasize the pervasiveness of health promotion and public health messages concerning "obesity." They demonstrate that despite different contexts, men and women around the globe are influenced by this discourse and the specific messages they receive about health. Such studies bring awareness of the different discourses that are drawn on when talking about bodies, what they should look like and feel like; they also highlight the effects of these discourses on health and bodily practices, the ways in which they influence daily bodily regimes, and subscription to a consumerist culture.

Method

Theoretical framework

We adopted a feminist poststructuralist framework largely informed by the writings of Weedon (1987, 1997), Gavey (1989), and Baxter (2003). Researchers adopting such a lens pay particular attention to issues of knowledge, power, language, and discourse, and how these intersect in the lives of women. Feminist poststructuralism offers an understanding of women's embodied experiences and their meanings (Currie 1999). It acknowledges the complex ways that meaning, institutions, power, subjectivity, and gender come together and allows for an explanation of the ways that sociocultural influences inform dominant practices (Kenway et al. 1994). The current study explores Jamaican women's accounts of their embodied experiences, particularly as they relate to health. Feminist poststructuralism allows for an explanation that considers their culture, gender, and class among other features.

Participants

Forty-one semistructured interviews were conducted with women from the Kingston/St. Andrew region of Jamaica. During the months of May to June 2015, the first author spoke with urban Jamaican women about their understandings of health and beauty and related bodily practices. Participants ranged in age from 18 to 62 years old, with an average age of 27 years old. The majority of the women were Black/Afro-Caribbean ($n = 30$), with a mixed-race minority ($n = 11$).[1] Those who were mixed race had parents who were from different racial groups—for example, one parent Black and the other, White. Other groups included Black and Indian, Black and Chinese or White and Chinese (or mixtures of these groups). Participants were also from diverse occupational backgrounds: 20 of the 41 women were either full-time or part-time students (11 of whom were studying either medicine, nursing, pharmacy, or biomedical science), 17 had full-time jobs working for the government or private companies, two had part-time jobs as workers in the entertainment industry, and two were retired. A small sample of the women interviewed (five of the 41), had either taken part in one or more beauty pageants or had some experience in Jamaica's modeling industry. Participants were of varying sizes; some identified as slim, others used the term *fluffy/thick* to describe their appearance. A few participants referred to themselves as average size.

Recruitment and procedure

Participants were recruited through the use of snowball sampling and posted advertisements placed at two university campuses and a driving school. Women interested in participating in the study were asked to contact the researcher to schedule a time and place to conduct the interview. Consent forms were reviewed and completed before the interview. With the exception of two Skype interviews, all were conducted in person. The interviews lasted between 30 min and 2.5 hr and were recorded using two digital audio recorders. Participants were given a $200 JMD phone card in appreciation for their participation in the study. Ethics approval was obtained from both the University of the West Indies' and the University of Guelph's research ethics boards. Pseudonyms were assigned before analysis and are used throughout the paper.

Transcription and data analysis

The interviews were transcribed verbatim into Word documents. Once all 41 interviews were transcribed and verified, transcripts were uploaded into NVivo 10 software (QSR International, Melbourne, Australia) and were individually coded for talk related to notions of health. Multiple codes were created for each topic. Analytic notes were made during both the transcription and coding process as the transcripts were read and reread several times. Following the example of Abou-Rizk and Rail (2012, 2014)), Harper and Rail (2010), Rail (2012), and Rail and Lafrance (2009), all of whom have conducted similar research on discursive constructions of the body, we utilized two methods of analysis: a thematic analysis (Braun and Clarke 2006) and a feminist poststructuralist discourse analysis (Gavey 1989; Weedon 1997). The thematic analysis was conducted as a form of preliminary analysis to assess what the participants had to say about health, while the feminist poststructuralist discourse analysis was used to examine how the participants spoke about health. For example, the thematic analysis illustrated that the size of the body, the types of food one should consume and the types of activities one needed to engage in were all pertinent themes related to health. The feminist poststructuralist discourse analysis allowed for an understanding of which discourses were adopted and rejected when participants described their ideas about health and the body. In the next section, we show how the discourses identified were adopted or rejected by our participants.

Results

Our results are organized according to two dominant discourses we identified in the Jamaican cultural context. The first is the "obesity epidemic" discourse. We trace how elements of this discourse are reproduced by Jamaican women in line with characterizations of the discourse previously documented by scholars in other cultural contexts. We then identify a second dominant discourse which was drawn on extensively by our participants. In contrast to the "obesity epidemic" discourse, which has been identified globally, this second discourse is specific to the local cultural context. We call this the slim-thick healthy body discourse.

"Obesity epidemic" discourse

In this section, we show how some participants drew on aspects of the "obesity epidemic" discourse when discussing (a) health as a personal responsibility and (b) evaluations of health according to body size. In the following extracts, words and phrases demonstrating the reproduction of this discourse are presented in bold.

Health as a personal responsibility

Participants discussed both the activities that one should engage in to achieve health, as well as the dangers of not living an active lifestyle and being responsible for one's health. For example, Michelle (60 years old, retired school teacher, Black/Afro-Caribbean) describes the perils she attributes to those considered "overweight." Her response is geared toward those who do not take an active interest in their dietary and exercise practices, that is, those whose bodies do not physically demonstrate that they are active.

> Michelle: ... **once you're "overweight", it predispose you to, to those things**, and I'm talking about especially those persons whose **"overweight" is caused from what they eat and lack of exercise**, it predispose you to **those chronic diseases**, it gives yu [your] heart more work to do, your movement, you can't move as, as you used to, so you keep on storing all of this, this fat, most of **the food that you're eating, and the lack of exercise can lead to diabetes, pressure on the heart, pressure you, you have high blood pressure and heart problems, so it predispose** you to those things.

Here, Michelle draws on several elements of the "obesity epidemic" discourse to explain the dangers of not being responsible for one's health. Evident in much of her talk is the notion of risk; Michelle draws on the "obesity epidemic" discourse to position those who are "overweight" as being at an increased risk for early mortality. She distinguishes between two types of "overweight" people: those whose excess weight is caused by poor lifestyle choices and those whose weight is attributed to other causes. She positions the former as responsible for their increased weight and negligent about their bodies, an association that is commonly made within the "obesity epidemic" discourse. She provides further evidence of uptake when she lists the variety of health issues that may result from excess body fat, thereby linking fat with disease, comorbidities, and early death.

Michelle situates her response about "overweight" bodies within an argument about the many risks and predispositions associated with such body types. She establishes her argument by drawing on authoritative biomedical associations between weight and ill health. Furthermore, by saying "those persons" she distances herself from fat people, creating an us-versus-them dynamic, whereby "those persons" are considered unhealthy. Michelle demonstrates how the shape and size of one's body are often considered representative of one's health and bodily practices.

Several other participants mentioned that their judgments about people's health were based on the notion that personal lifestyle practices and habits contribute to one's size. Therefore, if someone is fat, their lifestyle practices contributed to the outcome. In talking about women's bodies in this way, participants often introduced the idea that each individual is responsible for their own health, weight, and lifestyle. For example, Tricia, (28 years old, nail technician, Black/Afro-Caribbean) in the following extract, justifies her assumptions by placing emphasis on health habits and practices that are often associated with uncontrolled lifestyle practices.

Tricia: You have to eat a certain type of food to put on weight like that, so you definitely know that, that you eating too much of the wrong type of food, that's why they put on so much weight, they doh [don't] watch what they eat, they just eat eat, eat, eat, eat. **Bad eating habits also makes yuh [you] gain weight**, as yuh [you] eat and yuh [you] go sleep, that makes yuh [you] gain weight because the body doh [doesn't] get a chance, it takes three hours to digest the food … Just like if yuh [you] walking on the road and yuh [you] **see a very, very fat woman, yuh gonna seh [say] she nuh [not] healthy, look how she big an' fat, she cya [cant] be healthy**. That's the first thing that ago [is going to] come to yuh [your] mind inuh [you know], **she cya [cant] control her eating, the people dem a go seh [the people are going to say] she eat too much that's why she big suh [she's so big]**.

Tricia's use of the phrase "put on weight like that" suggests that there are specific behaviors and practices that are linked with a particular size. She pairs eating specific foods (those considered bad for the body)—and too much of them—with a big body size. This pairing demonstrates that when individuals reach a particular size, it is assumed that they are engaging in health-compromising behaviors and practices. Drawing on aspects of the "obesity" epidemic discourse, that is, (a) the importance of body maintenance and control over one's dietary habits and bodily practices and (b) linking thinness with good health, and fatness with ill health, Tricia makes judgments about people's dietary patterns, eating habits, and lifestyle practices. She shows uptake of this discourse by positioning very fat individuals as lacking control over their urges, eating practices and patterns. When she says "*they doh [don't] watch what they eat, they just eat eat, eat, eat, eat,*" the repetition of the word *eat* suggests that very fat women cannot be healthy, especially if their size is a result of their own actions (i.e., constant eating).

Evaluations of health according to body size

Several participants made assumptions about people's health based on the size of their bodies. Additionally, they relied on notions of self-sufficiency and functionality to explain how they make value judgments about health. For some participants, notions of health and body size were interrelated, while others described them as separate concepts. Those who spoke about size and health as being interrelated often discussed body size as a marker or indicator of health. Dione (32 years old, attorney at law, Black/Afro-Caribbean) describes the various bodily indicators of health that she draws on when making personal assessments.

> I: If someone were to ask you what the term health means to you, what comes to mind?
>
> Dione: I guess great skin usually is an indicator for me…maybe it's a poor indicator but for me if you have great skin I feel like that walks hand in hand with great health. **If you're too fat I probably feel like you're not very healthy.** That's an indication of **poor diet and probably the consumption of the bad foods**, you know you have the good foods and the bad foods. **So fatness obviously is an indication of poor health.** Also, super skinniness, like if you're too skinny. Something might be going on, unless it's a choice. Some people do choose to.

In the extract, Dione draws on aspects of the "obesity" epidemic discourse to make her point. Her response shows uptake of one of the main features, that is, conflating ill health with fatness, and good health with thinness. She also associates fatness with poor dietary choices and the consumption of foods that are considered bad for the body. Additionally, by her use of the word "obviously," she positions her claim as factual and draws attention to the pervasiveness of such links between health and weight, implying that such associations are well established, well documented, and frequently taken up in contemporary discourses. Dione reinforces the common notion that fatness is an indication of not only poor health, but poor lifestyle choices. Her choice of words also draws attention to the difference in health judgments made for those who are slim versus those who are fat. We see where she is cautious about the associations made between skinniness and health. She notes that it is likely that someone who is very skinny could also be ill if they are "too skinny"; however, she introduces the concept of choice to make a distinction between skinniness due to health issues and skinniness due to personal choice, as there are individuals who actively make an effort to maintain a specific level of slimness.[2] This extract demonstrates how Dione draws on different aspects of the "obesity" epidemic discourse to reinforce associations made between thinness and health.

Slim-thick healthy body discourse

Although the "obesity" epidemic discourse had a strong bearing on some women's reported health beliefs and practices, some aspects of the discourse were also strongly rejected. For example, when asked to describe a healthy body, some women described a range of body types that were often more inclusive of thicker frames than thin ones. This range was also more inclusive generally compared with the ideal healthy body that is advertised in Western fitness and fashion magazines. Although some participants subscribed to the thin ideal, several cited bigger, thicker bodies as the ideal healthy body for Jamaican women; in these instances, participants drew on what we have called the slim-thick health body discourse. Central features of this discourse oppose core tenets of Western notions of health and the body, for example: (a) an appreciation and endorsement of thicker body types (with an emphasis on wide hips and large buttocks) and (b) an association of thinness with illness and thickness with good health, strength, and attractiveness.

The participants described their versions of a healthy body as average in size, and explained that this was representative of a body that is "not too fat and not too thin" but could be considered thick. Some participants used the term *slim-thick*[3] to refer to this particular ideal. Similar to the findings of Abou-Rizk and Rail's (2014) study with young Lebanese Canadian women, the Jamaican women's version of their ideal body type was often very similar to their version of what a healthy body looked like, both of which were described as thicker than the body types portrayed in Western media outlets.

Almost all participants spoke about their ideal body as being thicker than bodies typically depicted in mainstream media; however, most mentioned that their ideal body would be just as toned. The participants' constructions of their ideal healthy body seemed to be closely associated with a particular level of thickness and excluded very thin and skinny bodies from the range of what is desirable. In the following extract, Laura (23 years old, biomedical sciences student, identifies as 'thick,' Black/Afro-Caribbean) draws on the slim-thick healthy body discourse to describe the variety of body types that are considered healthy in Jamaica. Words and phrases demonstrating the reproduction of the slim-thick discourse are presented in bold.

> I: What about in Jamaica, do you think there is a specific healthy weight or a specific body type that is seen as healthy?
>
> Laura: Yeah I definitely feel like for Jamaica, **a bigger, ok, like a more rounded person would be more** – like when you compare to Canada, would be **more seen as healthy rather than a super skinny person**. That's just how I see it in Jamaica because **everybody seems to want to be more kinda rounded or curvy ish kinda** and that seems to be like okay, whereas **sometimes when you have an extra skinny person they might think that they are a little malnourished**

or something. But in Canada, I feel like everybody is on a slimmer side, not really skinny but on a slimmer side more so than, more rounded or so. At least for most of the people, some of the minorities are more rounded but for the average day to day person, I think the slimmer side would be more seen as healthy as opposed to a more rounded person who would be considered like fat or chubby. So for Jamaica, **I would definitely say the rounded version seems to be more healthy**.

Laura, who spent some time in Canada for schooling, shares her observation on the difference in what is seen as a healthy weight in Jamaica versus in Canada. Drawing on the slim-thick healthy body discourse, she suggests that a curvier, more rounded figure is deemed healthy in Jamaica, while bodies that are slimmer are often thought to be malnourished. Unlike the "obesity" epidemic discourse that associates health with thinness, the slim-thick healthy body discourse evident in this extract links thinness with ill health and malnourishment.

In some instances, notions of health and beauty intersected, whereby participants spoke of fatness and thickness as both healthy and beautiful. Abigail (25 years old, customer service representative, Black/Afro-Caribbean) describes this intersection when asked how fatness is viewed in Jamaica.

Abigail: Umm, they think that **fat people are beautiful**, because they say that they're healthy, round and in colloquial terms, they would say that **"dem (they) look fat and nice"**

I: Okay.

Abigail: You know, so that is like, **big bottom, wide hips, big breasts. They wouldn't say that about slimmer girls you know, either them (they) have some disease or them (they) have AIDS or something or you know**, or just bones, stuff like that. They rather glorify bigger body type women.

Abigail describes the cultural endorsement of fatness in Jamaica. She reports the specific features of a woman's body that are valued in this context. Drawing on the slim-thick healthy body discourse, Abigail very clearly makes links between size and health, she notes that thinness is associated with very specific illnesses in the Jamaican context (e.g., AIDS), and emphasizes that bigger, thicker bodies tend to be culturally appreciated.

Summary of findings

There were notable trends in how the participants oriented themselves to the discourses. For example, participants positioned themselves as subjects based on how health was being discussed. When talking about health practices, the majority of participants reproduced aspects of the "obesity" discourse, that is, the importance of being active, eating well, and being self-sufficient. However, when asked if health had a particular look, a resistant subject position was often taken up to argue that a range of bodies could be classified as healthy. In our conversations, participants often navigated the two discourses to highlight these salient points. While some may not have taken up this discourse to position their own bodies, when talking about health within the Jamaican cultural context, all participants reproduced the slim-thick discourse to describe the Jamaican cultural ideal.

Discussion

The objective of this study was to describe how fatness is understood in Jamaica and identify the discourses that are available to urban Jamaican women. As with other studies (Abou-Rizk and Rail 2014; Pearce, Dibb, and Gaines 2014), the women in our study described their ideal "healthy" body as one that is not too fat and not too thin, bordering on "average" size. In a similar manner to the Lebanese Canadian women in Abou-Rizk and Rail's study, our participants argued that the thin frame depicted in fashion magazines is unrealistic, unhealthy and unattractive. Our findings support Gentles-Peart's (2013) study, suggesting that perhaps it is a Caribbean/ "West Indian thing" to find larger/thicker bodies healthy and attractive.

Our results confirmed previous findings (Pearce, Dibb, and Gaines 2014; Sobo 1993), that fatness tends to be viewed positively and is widely accepted in Jamaica. Our analysis also showed how powerful health discourses are in shaping the participants' understandings of health and the ways in which their bodies and subjectivities are constituted. As Wright (2009) argued, discourses pertaining to "obesity" and health are "the most powerful and pervasive discourses currently influencing ways of thinking about health and about bodies" (1). These discourses demonstrate how knowledge forms intersect and interact with each other to produce different ways of understanding the body.

Health and fitness discourses often constitute strong imperatives for how individuals should think, act, and feel about their bodies (Burrows, Wright, and Jungersen-Smith 2002). Given the pervasiveness of the "obesity" epidemic discourse globally, it was not surprising that several aspects were reproduced by the participants. Barned (2017) argued that the participant's reproduction of the "obesity" discourse is evidence of the circulation of commodified knowledges emanating from former colonizers and from hegemonic knowledge systems in the Anglo world. The circulation of such knowledge systems outside of their originating countries, whereby different cultural groups come to understand and regulate their bodies through rigid techniques of control and surveillance, is a form of neocolonialism. The Jamaican women's rearticulation of specific tenets of this discourse suggests that the values and ideals of former colonizers still have a powerful effect on the way of life of Jamaicans.

Critical theorists such as Huygens (2009) and Said (1988) examined the impact of "cultural ideologies, or systems of ideals, in creating and sustaining colonization and globalization" (Huygens 2009, 272). They argued that the production of cultural knowledge and the importance of maintaining Eurocentric ideals and an "unrelenting Eurocentrism" was one among many political and economic impetuses of colonization (Huygens 2009, 272; Said 1988, 294). According to Huygens, two specific ideologies were developed to naturalize European colonial expansion: colonial racism and European cultural supremacy. The establishment and success of these two ideologies would create a global culture and economy. We argue that the Jamaican women's reproduction of the "obesity" discourse highlights the success of European cultural supremacy and demonstrates how accessible European knowledge systems are.

The need for alternative discourses

In addition to the "obesity" epidemic discourse, the women in this study drew extensively on a local discourse, which we have called the slim-thick healthy body discourse. Our results suggest that this discourse was beneficial when describing a broader, more inclusive definition of health as it provided women with an alternative way of reading and making sense of their bodies and the bodies of others. Although the slim-thick healthy body discourse is more inclusive of bigger bodies, it is not without issue. One aspect of the discourse that is concerning is the labeling of very thin bodies as unhealthy or malnourished. This labeling positions thin bodies as abject. The present study therefore acknowledges the need for discourses that are inclusive of bodies on both ends of the weight continuum.

For curvy, voluptuous women, the slim-thick healthy body discourse makes available alternative ways of seeing oneself and one's body, and provides Jamaican women with an avenue of expression that does not center on slimness and body surveillance. For very thin women, the slim-thick healthy body discourse, similar to the "obesity" epidemic discourse, encourages body comparison and could possibly lead to feelings of inadequacy with one's size. This study suggests that the discourses that currently circulate in urban Jamaica are limited and constraining. There is therefore a need for alternative discourses (discourses that are more inclusive of bodies on either end of the weight spectrum) to provide Jamaican women with alternative subjectivities, and different ways of seeing themselves. The findings suggest that discourses that work to empower and uplift rather than shame and guilt are needed.

Critical health researchers and fat activists have discussed the potential of reclaiming fat identity by demedicalizing and reconceptualizing fatness and its associated meanings. They have called for alternative discourses around health and the body (Beausoleil and Ward 2010; Braziel and LeBesco 2001; LeBesco 2004), positing that if we think of fat as political and fat bodies as revolting against Western ideals of health and beauty, then we have made the first step toward reclaiming fat lives (LeBesco 2001). The slim-thick healthy body discourse is one such discourse that attends to these issues. One of the most popular body messages perpetuated by many is that people need to be thin to be healthy. We agree that health should not be assessed by the size of one's body; less emphasis needs to be placed on health at one size (i.e., thinness) and more on the many different forms and looks that health could have. As Rail (2010) noted,

> we must worry about the recitation of a discourse that emphasizes the importance of 'not being fat' and having a 'normal' body as such discourse is particularly oppressive to corpulent or physically disabled youth whose bodies are often constructed in opposition to 'normality' and 'health.' (150)

The slim-thick healthy body discourse endorses body diversity (to an extent) and posits specifically that there is a range of body types that are considered healthy. For racialized women, such a discourse opens up avenues to embrace values that are different from the Euro-American norm. Our findings suggest that people from Non-Western cultural groups draw on their own understandings of health, further confirming that some racialized women understand their bodies in ways that align with their cultural background. It is clear that we need to be more critical of our understandings of health and the body types that constitute health. A critical assessment would allow individuals to effectively disentangle definitions and depictions of health that are based on Euro-American standards (i.e., thin) from more diverse and inclusive depictions (health at a variety of sizes).

Challenging and changing dominant discourses in Jamaica

Challenging and changing dominant health discourses is not easily achieved. However, we suggest two possible avenues to facilitate change in Jamaica. These include body positive campaigns and social media intervention. Body positive campaigns endorsed by Jamaica's Ministry of Health and Ministry of Education that introduce more inclusive ways of talking about bodies may be an effective way to influence dominant discourses. Such campaigns could target the general population and promote the concept of health in varying shapes and sizes. In an effort to be more inclusive than the discourses that already exist, these campaigns would also need to approach issues of weight from multiple perspectives (i.e., not privileging a biomedical approach).

Launching such a campaign through key social media figures in Jamaica would ensure a wide reach among the Jamaican population. Popular emcee and social media figures, Miss Kitty, and Yanique the "curvy" diva, both have very large social media followings on Instagram and Facebook. Although users of these social media platforms vary by age, and may be associated with younger generations, launching such campaigns with the help of these women would contribute significantly toward changing the ways people talk about health and fatness. Through local radio and TV shows, Miss Kitty and Yanique have both spoken about their experiences living in bodies that are considered thicker than average. Both have discussed their attempts at reclaiming how people read their bodies, and have positively impacted how fatness is understood in Jamaica. Miss Kitty's slogan of "fluffy, fabulous and fit" encourages women to embrace one's size (The Gleaner 2013), and could be interpreted as a local manifestation of fat activism. It is likely that due to their prior body positive associations, messages addressing inclusive ways of discussing health and beauty may be well received if coming from them. Our findings suggest that there is indeed a need for alternative ways of talking about bodies. Addressing this need may help efforts toward a movement of self-acceptance, self-love, and body positivity in Jamaica.

Conclusion

Being big-bodied is often paired with experiences of prejudice, negative stereo-types, and low self-esteem. The slim-thick healthy body discourse creates a safe space for big-bodied women to feel empowered in their bodies, in that labelling oneself as thick, slim-thick, or fluffy provides women with a mechanism that preserves their self-esteem and self-worth (Barned and Lipps 2014). Here, we argue that health can be achieved in different ways; our findings suggest that women of racialized backgrounds achieve their own versions of health by means of diversifying what health looks like. The Jamaican women in our study created a space for themselves outside dominant Euro-American standards, where they can reclaim their bodies as both healthy and beautiful.

Notes

1 Throughout the results, we position the participants in varied ways. The inconsistent positioning of participants (e.g., in terms of age, body size, and skin color) is largely due to the fact that demographics were not collected during data collection; as a result, the identifiers used are based on how participants described themselves throughout conversations with the researcher.
2 As might models or beauty pageant contestants.
3 This term is commonly used in Jamaica to refer to bodies that are on the thicker side.

References

Abou-Rizk, Z., and G. Rail. 2012. ""Disgusting" Fat Bodies & Young Lebanese-Canadian Women's Discursive Constructions of Health." *Women's Health & Urban Life* 11 (1):94–123.

Abou-Rizk, Z., and G. Rail. 2014. ""Judging a Body by Its Cover": Young Lebanese-Canadian Women's Discursive Constructions of the "Healthy" Body and "Health" Practices." *Journal of Immigrant and Minority Health* 16 (1):150–64. doi:10.1007/s10903-012-9757-5.

Anderson-Fye, E. P. 2004. "A "Coca-Cola" Shape: Cultural Change, Body Image, and Eating Disorders in San Andres, Belize." *Culture, Medicine and Psychiatry* 28 (4):561–95.

Barned, C. (2017). *"Not fat, maybe thick, not too skinny": Resisting and reproducing health and beauty discourses in urban Jamaica* (Doctoral dissertation). Retrieved from The Atrium, University of Guelph. http://hdl.handle.net/10214/11425

Barned, C., and G. E. Lipps. 2014. "Development and Validation of a Measure of Attitudes toward Fluffy Women." *The West Indian Medical Journal* 63 (6):626.

Baxter, J. 2003. *Positioning Gender in Discourse.* New York, NY: Palgrave Macmillan.

Beausoleil, N., and P. Ward. 2010. "Fat Panic in Canadian Public Health Policy: Obesity as Dif- Ferent and Unhealthy." *Radical Psychology* 8:1.

Braun, V., and V. Clarke. 2006. "Using Thematic Analysis in Psychology." *Qualitative Research in Psychology* 3 (2):77–101. doi:10.1191/1478088706qp063oa.

Braziel, J. E., and K. LeBesco (Eds.). 2001. *Bodies Out of Bounds: Fatness and Transgression.* London, England: Univ of California Press.

Burrows, L., J. Wright, and J. Jungersen-Smith. 2002. ""Measure Your Belly": New Zealand Children's Constructions of Health and Fitness." *Journal of Teaching in Physical Education* 22: 39–48. doi: 10.1123/jtpe.22.1.39.

Currie, D.H. 1999. *Girl Talk: Adolescent Magazines and Their Readers.* Toronto: University of Toronto Press.

Gard, M., and D. Kirk. 2007. "Obesity Discourse and the Crisis of Faith in Disciplinary Technology." *Utibildning & Demokrati* 16 (2):17–36.

Gard, M., and J. Wright. 2005. *The Obesity Epidemic: Science, Morality and Ideology.* London, England: Routledge.

Gavey, N. 1989. "Feminist Poststructuralism and Discourse Analysis: Contributions to Feminist Psychology." *Psychology of Women Quarterly* 13: 459–75. doi: 10.1111/j.1471-6402.1989.tb01014.x.

Gentles-Peart, K. 2013. "West Indian Immigrant Women, Body Politics, and Cultural Citizenship." In *Bodies Without Borders*, edited by de Casanova E.M., Jafar A., 25–43. New York, US: Palgrave Macmillan.

George, T., and G. Rail. 2006. "Barbie Meets the Bindi: Constructions of Health among Second Generation South Asian Canadian Women." *Journal of Women's Health & Urban Life* 4 (2):45–67.

Grindley, L. 2013, July 28. Fluffy, Fabulous and Fit. *The Jamaica Gleaner*. http://jamaica-gleaner.com/gleaner/20130728/out/out1.html

Harper, E. A., and G. Rail. 2010. "Contesting "Silhouettes of a Pregnant Belly": Young Pregnant Women's Discursive Constructions of the Body." *Aporia* 1 (3):5–14.

Hobson, J. 2003. "The "Batty" Politic: Toward an Aesthetic of the Black Female Body." *Hypatia* 18 (4):87–105.

Huygens, I. 2009. "From Colonization to Globalization: Continuities in Colonial 'Commonsense'." In *Introduction to Critical Psychology*, 2nd ed., 267–84, London, England: Sage. ISBN 9781847871732.

Jafar, A., and E. Casanova (Eds.). 2013. *Global Beauty, Local Bodies*. New York, NY.: Palgrave McMillian.

Kenway, J., S. Willis, J. Blackmore, and L. Rennie. 1994. "Making "Hope Practical" Rather than "Despair Convincing": Feminist Poststructuralism, Gender Reform and Educational Change." *British Journal of Sociology and Education* 15: 187–210. doi: 10.1080/0142569940150203.

Kwan, S., and J. Graves. 2013. *Framing Fat: Competing Constructions in Contemporary Culture*. New Brunswick, New Jersey: Rutgers University Press.

Lawrence, R.G. 2004. "Framing Obesity: The Evolution of News Discourse on a Public Health Issue." *Harvard International Journal of Press/Politics* 9 (3):56–75. doi:10.1177/1081180X04266581.

LeBesco, K. 2001. "Revolting Bodies: The Resignification of Fat in Cyber Space." In *Technospaces. Inside the New Media*, edited by S. R. Munt, 175–88. London and New York: Continuum.

LeBesco, K. 2004. *Revolting Bodies: The Struggle to Redefine Fat Identity*. Amherst, MA: University of Massachusetts Press.

Miller, E. L. 1969. "Body Image, Physical Beauty and Color among Jamaican Adolescents." *Social and Economic Studies* 18 (1):72–89.

Mohammed, P. 2000. "" But Most of All Mi Love Me Browning": The Emergence in Eighteenth and Nineteenth-Century Jamaica of the Mulatto Woman as the Desired'." *Feminist Review* 65 (Summer):22–48. doi:10.1080/014177800406921.

Patton, T. O. 2006. "Hey Girl, Am I More than My Hair?: African American Women and Their Struggles with Beauty, Body Image, and Hair." *NWSA Journal* 18 (2):24–51. doi:10.2979/nws.2006.18.issue-2.

Pearce, V., B. Dibb, and S. O. Gaines Jr. 2014. "Body Weight Perceptions, Obesity and Health Behaviours in Jamaica." *Caribbean Journal of Psychology* 6 (1):43–61.

Rail, G. 2010. "Canadian Youth's Discursive Constructions of Health in the Context of Obesity Discourse." In *Biopolitics and the Obesity Epidemic*, edited by J. Wright and V. Harwood, 141–56. New York and London: Routeledge.

Rail, G. 2012. "The Birth of the Obesity Clinic: Confessions of the Flesh, Biopedagogies and Physical Culture." *Sociology of Sport Journal* 29 (1):227–53. doi:10.1123/ssj.29.2.227.

Rail, G., D. Holmes, and S. J. Murray. 2010. "The Politics of Evidence on 'Domestic Terrorists': Obesity Discourses and Their Effects." *Social Theory & Health* 8 (3):259–79. doi:10.1057/sth.2009.10.

Rail, G., and M. Lafrance. 2009. "Confessions of the Flesh and Biopedagogies: Discursive Constructions of Obesity on Nip/Tuck." *Medical Humanities* 35 (2):76–79. doi:10.1136/jmh.2009.001610.

Rice, C. 2014. *Becoming Women: The Embodied Self in Image Culture*. Toronto: University of Toronto Press.

Rich, E., and J. Evans. 2005. "'Fat Ethics'– The Obesity Discourse and Body Politics." *Social Theory & Health* 3 (4):341–58. doi:10.1057/palgrave.sth.8700057.

Said, E. W. 1988. *Nationalism, Colonialism and Literature: Yeats and Decolonization*. vol. 15. Derry, Ireland: Field Day.

Savacool, J. 2009. *The World Has Curves: The Global Quest for the Perfect Body*. New York: Rodale Books.

Sobo, E. J. 1993. *One Blood: The Jamaican Body*. Albany, NY: State University of New York (SUNY) Press.

Tate, S. 2007. "Black Beauty: Shade, Hair and Anti-Racist Aesthetics." *Ethnic and Racial Studies* 30 (2):300–19. doi:10.1080/01419870601143992.

Tate, S. 2013. "The Performativity of Black Beauty Shame in Jamaica and Its Diaspora: Problematizing and Transforming Beauty Iconicities." *Feminist Theory* 14 (2):219–35. doi:10.1177/1464700113483250.

Tull, E. S., C. Butler, T. Wickramasuriya, H. Fraser, E. C. Chambers, V. Brock, … E. Haney. 2001. "Should Body Size Preference Be a Target of Health Promotion Efforts to Address the Epidemic of Obesity in Afro-Caribbean Women?" *Ethnicity & Disease* 11 (4):652–60.

Weedon, C. 1987. *Feminist Practice & Poststructuralist Theory*. Oxford: Basil Blackwell Ltd.

Weedon, C. 1997. *Feminist Practice & Poststructuralist Theory*, 2nd ed. Oxford: Blackwell.

Wilk, R. 1995. "The Local and the Global in the Political Economy of Beauty: From Miss Belize to Miss World." *Review of International Political Economy* 2 (1):117–34. doi:10.1080/09692299508434312.

Wright, J. 2009. "Biopower, Biopedagogies and the Obesity Epidemic." In *Biopolitics and the 'Obesity Epidemic': Governing Bodies*, edited by J. Wright and V. Harwood, 1–14. London and New York: Routeldge.

Wright, J., G. O'Flynn, and D. Macdonald. 2006. "Being Fit and Looking Healthy: Young Women's and Men's Constructions of Health and Fitness." *Sex Roles* 54 (9–10):707–16. doi:10.1007/s11199-006-9036-9.

Frozen: A fat tale of immigration

Cat Pausé

ABSTRACT

Fat people are constructed as failed citizens; they are believed to be a burden on society, consuming too many resources and costing too many healthcare monies. In modern neoliberal contexts, this results in hostile environments and the development of spoiled identities (stigmatized identities in which the bearer is held responsible for the stigma). These hostile environments are demonstrated in many ways: governments failing to designate weight as a category protected from discrimination, public health campaigns aimed at battling the "war on obesity," and immigration policies that exclude people based on body mass index. The author explores the latter using an autoethnographic method; the author, who was excluded from obtaining a resident visa in New Zealand because of her body mass index, uses her personal experiences battling an immigration system to explore these biopolitics and their role in (re) producing fat oppression.

> The medical assessor has advised that you do not meet the acceptable standard of health for entry to New Zealand on the basis that you are likely to impose significant costs or demands on New Zealand's health services. (Letter from Immigration New Zealand, July 1, 2010)

This line, in a letter from Immigration New Zealand, informed me that my application for a resident visa was likely to be denied because I had failed to meet the acceptable standard of health. In reading further into the letter, it became clear that the acceptable standard of health I had failed to meet was having an appropriate body mass index (BMI). In short, New Zealand didn't want me because I was too fat.

In previous work, I have briefly discussed the frustration and shame I experienced from being denied residency in New Zealand based on my BMI (Lee and Pausé 2016). In this piece, I delve deeper, bringing the reader through the process I underwent for Immigration New Zealand; the many hoops through which I had to jump, the biases I had to overcome, and the feelings of shame I had to negotiate. I do this to illuminate how the mechanisms of the State operate to oppress fat people through immigration policies and procedures, denying fat people opportunities to work and reside in countries around the world. I've used autoethnography, which allows me to share my personal experiences and feelings through a lens of theory and literature to construct meaning and develop theory (Ellis, Adams, and Bochner 2011).

Autoethnography is especially useful for developing new theories and building the literature of emerging disciplines of scholarship; many fat studies scholars have found it a useful methodology in their work (Cooper 2016; Lee and Pausé 2016). For example, Murray (2005) and Pausé (2012a) used autoethnography to explore fat identity management and ambivalence. Autoethnography allows the scholar to study and reflect on their own experiences to inform scholarship; using lived experience as data has been integral in the discipline of fat studies, as voices and experiences of fat people are rarely included in mainstream "obesity" and weight research. Centering the experiences of fat people is a hallmark characteristic of fat studies scholarship.

Rinaldi et al. (2017) suggested that body size has been undertheorized in relation to citizenship. Bacchi and Beasley (2002) noted that scholarship on bodies (or embodiment) and citizenship have rarely intersected. They suggested that this gap is best explained by the distance between the public (citizenship) and the private (bodies). But this distance can only be observed for bodies that are normative and carry privilege (White bodies, male bodies, abled bodies, non-fat bodies, etc.). Other bodies, including bodies of color, bodies with disabilities, and fat bodies, have long been positioned as public concerns and sites of surveillance, legislation, and regulation. The intersection of bodies and citizenship within Western societies have been especially strong since the Second World War, when connections were strongly made between healthy ("fit") bodies and the workforce required to uphold democracy and build the wealth of the middle classes in the Global North (Elliott 2007). As Global North societies have moved away from physical labor economies to technology economies, the concerns with fatness have been reframed to economic costs, rather than labor costs (Elliott 2007). In 2001, U.S. Surgeon General David Satcher stood alongside the Department of Health and Human Services Secretary Tommy Thompson and announced "all Americans – as part of their patriotic duty – [should] lose 10 pounds" (Herndon 2005, 128). Fat bodies are positioned as unpatriotic because they represent an unnecessary strain on the healthcare system, a burden on their fellow citizens (Herndon 2005). These arguments are all components of a larger understanding of biopolitics, a term from Foucault (1990) that encompasses the range of activities associated with political power and its relationship with the bodies of any given population. For fat people, biopolitics can be plainly seen in government attempts to surveil, legislate, and regulate, fat bodies. Harjunen (2016) suggested that biopolitical actions can be best understood as a tool of neoliberalism, an idea taken up later in this piece.

My experiences with immigrating to a new country were precipitated by accepting an academic position at Massey University in New Zealand. To legally work in the country, I applied for a Work to Residence visa before leaving my home country of the United States. The website of Immigration New Zealand guides those interested in coming to New Zealand through interactive tools that inform them of their options for entering New Zealand (Immigration New Zealand, "Welcome").

I was especially interested in whether my weight would be a barrier to emigrating, as I had heard horror stories online from other fat people who found themselves denied visas to countries in the Global North. A requirement for any visa in New Zealand is to meet the "health and character requirements". The health requirements are identified as such on the Immigration New Zealand website (Immigration New Zealand, "Health"):

To come to New Zealand you must have an acceptable standard of health, or be granted a medical waiver. We'll consider you have an acceptable standard of health if you're:

- unlikely to be a danger to the health of the people already in New Zealand
- unlikely to cost New Zealand's health or special education services a lot of money
- able to work or study if this the [sic] reason for your visa.

This didn't seem to bode well for me from the start. While there didn't appear to be an explicit criteria regarding a BMI cutoff, I could easily imagine that having a high BMI would be considered something that may be costly. Luckily, I was able to secure a two-year Work to Residence visa. And while this visa would normally make me automatically eligible for residency after two years of employment, mine was flagged due to my "morbid obesity"; further review of my "condition" would be required before additional visas would be granted. The story I share here is my journey to gain a resident visa, which would allow me the right to live and work in New Zealand indefinitely.

Immigration New Zealand policy is set within the larger framework of neoliberalism that guides New Zealand governance. Neoliberalism systems seek to uncouple the state for any responsibility for the health and well-being of their citizens; it is up to individuals to look after themselves (Harjunen 2016; LeBesco 2011). Individual decisions regarding self-surveillance, self-governance, and health-seeking behaviors determine whether an individual is regarded as a responsible citizen. Irresponsible citizens are those that make decisions that ultimately may (will) place undue burden on the state (Pausé 2015). Fat people have been identified as a group that is responsible for great costs to society (Elliott 2007; Swinburn et al. 1997); "in quantifiable terms, the fat citizen is a failing citizen, their costs outweighing their contributions" (Rinaldi et al. 2017, 221). This echoes the theorizing of fat bodies as failed subjects by Murray (2005), who suggested that fat bodies are known to be weak and out of control. Fat bodies are lazy bodies, and their laziness costs society. These costs are made concrete through suggestions of fat people being less productive in their jobs than their non-fat colleagues, and requiring more healthcare resources than their non-fat friends and family.

For anyone intending to stay in New Zealand for more than 12 months, a medical certificate must be completed to provide "evidence you're in good health" (Immigration New Zealand, "Health"). On the General Medical Certificate, the first sentence reads, "Applicants for entry to New Zealand are required to have an acceptable standard of health" (Immigration New Zealand 2016). The document then continues to explain the responsibilities of the applicant, what they will need to supply to the physician when they attend their appointment, and what to expect when they see a physician to complete the certificate.

In Section C of the General Medical Certification, the applicant is required to declare that the information provided is true, complete, and correct. They sign that they "understand that [their] personal details and health information are being collected to enable Immigration New Zealand, Ministry of Business, Innovation, and Employment, to determine whether or not they are satisfied that [the applicant] meet the health criteria for a New Zealand visa" (Immigration New Zealand 2016, 7). Rinaldi et al. (2017) highlighted the important role that the medical community plays in identifying good and bad citizens; "medical practitioners are prescribing and inscribing technologies of self, and are playing a role in the production of a particular biocitizenry" (223). New Zealand has delegated the responsibility of determining good and bad potential citizens, based on health status and potential health risks, to the Ministry of Health. The Ministry, in turn, identifies health requirements necessary for entry into New Zealand.

Round 1

I engaged my regular physician to help me complete the medical certificate. Within the physical examination, the second and third questions relate to the applicant's height and weight, allowing for the calculation of the answer for question four: BMI. Toward the end of the section, the physician is asked to identity whether there are "any physical or mental conditions which may prevent this person from attending a mainstream school, gaining full employment or living independently now or in the future" (Immigration New Zealand 2016, 10). This is the first opportunity for a member of the medical community to alert Immigration New Zealand that a person may be an unappealing addition, draining more from society than they are contributing.

Within my medical certificate, the physician noted my "abnormal" appearance of "obesity," but noted there were no conditions that might affect my "ability to earn a living, attend a mainstream school, take care of [myself] or adapt to a new environment now or in future adult life" (Immigration New Zealand 2016, 10). It also noted that my completed urine and blood tests (both standard and discretionary) were within normal limits. Medical certificate in hand, I completed the remaining requirements and submitted my visa application.

Round 2

A few months later, in May 2010, I received a letter from immigration sharing that the Immigration New Zealand medical assessor needed more information before proceeding, including additional blood tests, a report from an endocrinologist, and the answers to the following questions, "What is the cause [of the obesity]? Is there target organ damage present? Is bariatric surgery recommended? What is the prognosis?"

The assessor wanted to know the cause of my fatness and the prognosis. My fatness had obviously been problematized, and more specifically, pathologized. "Obesity" was designated as a disease by the American Medical Association in 2013 (Pollack 2013), and many government health organizations around the Western world took up the designation soon after. Jutel (2006) argued that "a state which might otherwise have been seen as simply bothersome or irritating takes on a new significance when it becomes a diagnosis" (2268). Some fat people believe the disease designation for "obesity" will allow for better treatment protocols and the decrease of stigma associated with fatness, while others believe it to be yet another way to oppress fat people (Pausé 2014). Critical scholars have long argued that the positioning of "obesity" as a public health crisis is based on assumptions about the relationship between weight and health that have limited evidentiary support (e.g., Campos et al. 2005). As both a fat studies scholar and fat activist, I do not support the classification that my body is diseased. In fact, I find it offensive that I am a disease that many are seeking to cure. However, my personal feelings had no bearing on the requirements of Immigration New Zealand. If I wanted to continue working in New Zealand, I needed to follow their prescribed protocol.

The endocrinologist

To see an endocrinologist, I had to see another general practitioner to get a referral. Rather than returning to the doctor who completed my initial medical certificate, I sought out a new doctor. I asked around to see if I could find a doctor who might work from a Health At Every Size (HAES) perspective. I called the local women's center, which keeps records on healthcare providers for just such a purpose, but was disappointed to learn that attitudes around body size and treatment of fat people hadn't been something they had collected data on previously. I encouraged them to begin including this whenever possible. I ended up seeing a relatively young expat at a practice in a low socioeconomic part of town. Before my initial appointment, I wrote him a letter, explaining the circumstances of the appointment, along with my own perspective on the questions being asked by the Immigration New Zealand medical assessor. My appointment with the general practitioner (GP) went very well. While uneducated on HAES himself, he was very receptive to the tenets of the philosophy.

Referral in hand, I made an appointment with the only endocrinologist in town. While I waited, I wrote and sent him a letter, explaining the circumstances of the appointment, along with my own perspective on the questions being asked by the Immigration New Zealand medical assessor. In this letter, I included the following paragraph:

> I appreciate that the medical board would like further review by you to explore my health and endocrine system. I reject, however, any assumption that my weight is a good predictor of my health, or that being 'deathly fat' is, in itself, unhealthy. I reject these assumptions based on my knowledge of obesity research, epidemiology, and fat studies. I am a fat studies academic, and I work to unpack the obesity myth and to increase fat acceptance across Aotearoa, New Zealand.

My visit with the endocrinologist was a nightmare from start to finish. As I waited for the doctor to see me, I chatted with his wife. She was incredulous to my belief that being fat wasn't an indicator of poor health, and unsympathetic to my concern at being denied residency based on my weight. As a precursor to my time with her husband, it was prescient. He had already completed much of the exam paperwork before I had entered the room. His practice was unable to accommodate my large body; the gown was too small, the blood pressure cuff as well. He didn't ask any questions about my health behaviors, my health history, or my family health history. I offered up evidence of my good fatty performance (Bias 2014), my nutritious diet, avoidance of fast food, and regular exercise routine.

He did listen to my heart, check my reflexes, and palpate my abdomen. There was obvious discomfort on his part in the latter; I was extremely uncomfortable as well, having someone obviously not interested in providing care to a fat body like mine, touch me in such an intimate way. I couldn't remember the last time someone had touched my belly. After I re-dressed, he dismissed my within range/limits blood tests, assuring me that my size would catch up with me as I aged, and I'd be diabetic before I was thirty. I left his practice feeling devastated, shamed, and sullied.

He provided a letter for Immigration New Zealand that addressed the questions posed. He also included some information about hazard ratios related to having a BMI above 40, concluding "Because of her lack of other risk factors and the fact that she has a reasonably healthy diet and exercises regularly may well significantly modify these hazard ratios." If I had not shared with him information about my dietary intake and exercise routine would his conclusion have changed? And what role did my letter sent beforehand make? Other fat activists and scholars have suggested that presenting a letter to a new doctor can reduce the anxiety felt by fat people who have a history of received biased and discriminatory care from healthcare professionals. Hanne Blank ("Letter to a doctor", n.d), for example, provides an example of a letter that she provided when she began with a new GP.

Round 3

A month after my appointment with the endocrinologist, I received the decision. The Immigration New Zealand medical assessor had determined that I did not meet the "acceptable standard of health for entry to New Zealand on the basis that [I] am likely to impose significant costs or demands on New Zealand's health services"; this significant cost is quantified in the judgement as "costing in excess of NZ$25,000." From the medical assessor's judgement,

> The applicant is morbidly obese ... this is not consistent with long term health given the increased future risk of diabetes, cancer, ischaemic heart disease ... given the applicant is young the applicant has not yet developed any overt complications of her obesity to date. However over time this is highly likely and there is a relatively high probability of requiring health services in the future in relation to her gross morbid obesity ... there is a possibility that ability to work could be compromised due to gross obesity.

The letter concludes by informing me that I may provide additional information, including a second medical opinion, to be considered. I turned to the GP who had provided the referral to the endocrinologist, and he supplied a disputing medical opinion. In his letter to Immigration New Zealand, he noted that I was in "excellent health and [had] no health issues." He stated, "I see no objective health barriers as to why this lady should be refused immigration" and concluded, "Incidentally, her occupation is sedentary and her ability to work depends on her mental function rather than her physical function." I found this final sentence odd, although I guess technically accurate. My work as an academic requires me to engage in a great deal of thinking, reading, and writing, but asks very little from my physical body besides being awake and aware; this is especially true as most of my teaching takes place online as well.

I also supplied additional information in the form of a statement to the medical assessor(s). In my statement, I noted,

> I am writing this in response to notification that the medical assessor for NZ Immigration has determined that I do not meet the acceptable standards of health for permanent residency. As my medical tests and reports are all within normal ranges, this determination must be based solely on my BMI.

The medical opinion is that:

(1) There is a relatively high probability that the applicant's chronic recurring medical condition(s) over the course of the condition(s) will require health services costing in excess of NZ$25,000.
  - Response: I am unaware of what chronic recurring medical condition is being referred to. As the numerous medical tests requested by immigration demonstrate, I am in excellent health. I do not have a chronic recurring medical condition. Being fat is not a disease, any more than being thin is an indication of good health.
(2) This is not consistent with long term good health given the increased future risk of diabetes, cancer, ischaemic heart disease, osteo-arthritis, renal and respiratory disease, along with other medical conditions and morbidity.
  - Response: What evidence is this conclusion based on?
(3) Given the applicant is young, the applicant has not yet developed any overt complications of her obesity to date. However, over time, this is highly likely and there is a relatively high probability of requiring health services in the future in relation to her gross morbid obesity. Health services are already overburdened.
  - Response: As evidenced by my medical tests and examinations (by three separate physicians, including the endocrinologist), I am in good health. There is no reason to expect this to change. What evidence is the assessor basing their conclusion on?
(4) There is a possibility that ability to work could be compromised due to gross obesity.
  - Response: What evidence is this conclusion is based on? Also, there is always a possibility that a person's ability to work could be compromised due to ill health, accident, disability, or death, regardless of their BMI.

This was followed by a 12-page (!!!) paper that explored the empirical literature on the BMI, the relationship between weight and health, and the efficacy of weight loss. It was supported by nine additional pages of references, drawing largely from empirical journals such as the *Journal of the American Medical Association, New England Journal of Medicine, International Journal of Obesity, International Journal of Epidemiology*, and *Obesity Research*. I remember sharing this paper with others at the time, and most of them were gobsmacked at the amount of effort and time that would have been required to prepare the summary. I was asked, time and again, why so many references? Why such attention to detail? It was harder to explain then than it would be now, but the reason was because I felt as the failed subject (Murray 2005), I had to be EXTRA. Extra thorough. Extra scientific. Extra.

Whereas the endocrinologist didn't feel the need to include supporting evidence for his statements about hazard ratios, and the Immigration New Zealand medical assessor didn't feel the need to include supporting evidence for their statements about future costs or demands on New Zealand's health services predictions based on my BMI, I *did* feel the need to fully support my statements with empirical evidence. The reason for this was twofold. First, because my statements were not aligned with the dominant "obesity" discourses, I felt it necessary to support them with a preponderance of evidence. Second, because, as a fat person, I am always seen as suspect. I am not trusted to know truths about fatness, my own body, my own behaviors; fat people are not allowed to be producers of knowledge (Cooper 2016; Pausé 2012b). Doctors, especially, expect me to lie to them about my health behaviors and health status (Foster et al. 2003; Hebl and Xu 2001; Lee and Pausé 2016). When I argue for fat people having the same rights as non-fat people, my fat body reveals a secret motive I have for my activism. When I question the dominant "obesity" discourse, my fat body signifies my desire to provide a justification for my existence, or excuses for my size. My fat body speaks louder than I do.

The assessors

Three medical assessors for Immigration New Zealand considered the additional information. After that, all three produced reports and noted that I would likely impose significant costs or demands on New Zealand health services, including "publicly-funded health services for which the current demand is not being met." Fat bodies have long been constructed as impending sites of disease, and thereby, medical costs (e.g., Parker and Pausé 2018), and this was the primary factor identified by the medical assessors as to why I did not meet an acceptable standard of health. All three ticked the box that identified I was "likely to <u>impose significant costs or demands</u> on New Zealand's health services during their period of intended stay in New Zealand. There is a relatively high probability that the applicant's <u>chronic recurring medical condition(s)</u> over the course of the condition(s) will require health services costing in excess of NZ$25,000" (emphasis theirs). As noted by Assessor 1, "over time [overt complications of obesity are] highly likely and there is a relatively high probability of requiring health services in the future in relation to her gross morbid obesity." My fatness is a threat: a threat to me (through disease and early death), the State (through costs associated with "obesity"; see Swinburn et al. 1997), and even humanity (threatening the very survival of the human race, on par with global warming and weapons of mass destruction; e.g., Pace 2006).

And my current state of good health, as noted across the assessments (as well as the endocrinologist), was not seen as a protector to (or even consideration of) these future costs. My good health was considered a temporary state that would expire in the future because of my fatness. The endocrinologist told me, as he dismissed me from his office, that I would develop diabetes by age thirty. All three of the Immigration New Zealand medical assessors noted that my fat body was a ticking time-bomb. Assessor 2 noted that I was "presently in stable health – but is only 31 years of age"; they did not identify at which age I could expect my stable health to alter because of my weight. Assessor 1 stated that I was "young [therefore] there is relatively high probability that complications of [my] obesity will become evident over time," and Assessor 3 began their report by summarizing, "this woman has gross morbid obesity but as of yet has not developed any co-morbidities." All of the assessors made estimations about my future health based on my current body size. They were comfortable in predicting my health in the near and far future, based on their generalizations about my fatness. (Although I will give credit to Assessor 2, who did try to acknowledge the generalizing that was taking place, noting, "There are always exceptions to rules in medicine but we need to base our recommendations on probabilities and with a BMI of over 60 we would have to state that there is a relatively high probability of developing one or more of the medical complications associated with morbid obesity"). One assessor noted that bariatric surgery might be a useful preventative measure. Because of the belief that body size is mutable, fatness is understood as a condition that can be altered through discipline, willpower, or surgery. This is reinforced through exploitainment shows such as *The Biggest Loser* or *I Used to Be Fat* (Hass 2018), weight loss before/after photos (Fox 2018), and most fictional presentations of fatness in mainstream culture (Byers 2018).

The report provided by Assessor 3 was the most striking, both in tone and in presentation. The report was poorly structured, and lacking appropriate punctuation. There were several spelling and grammatical errors, and no coherent connections or transitions between sections. The assessor notes, with an underline to emphasize the statement, that I am "266% overweight." The assessor states that insurance companies use actuarial tables to assess risk associated with BMI, and provides a definition of "obesity" from the dictionary. The report suggests that "There are always Authors with contrary opinions available on the Internet but Medical Assessors are influenced by ! Their experiences 2. By peer review, and by access to respected textbooks and journals and 3. by Guidelines from the Immigration Department (INZ)" [sic]. And the report concludes by noting that "the consideration here is not being obese but groos morbis obesity ie this candidate would be uninsurable with a Life Insurance Company, Actuarial tables" (a handwritten correction was made to make "groos morbis obesity" to "gross morbid obesity"). If this had been work submitted by one of my students, it would have received a failing grade.

Assessor 3, along with their judgement, attached a selection of pages from the second edition of Brackenridge's (1985) *Medical Selection of Life Risks: A Comprehensive Guide to Life Expectancy for Underwriters and Clinicians*, the first page from Swinburn et al. (1997)'s "Health care costs of obesity in New Zealand," an illegible first page of "Body-mass index and cause-specific mortality in 900,000 adults: collaborative analyses of 57 prospective studies" (Prospective Studies Collaboration 2009) from the *Lancet*, and several additional pages of unknown origins on "obesity."

The rage I felt as I tried to read and understand the report from the third assessor was unrivalled in my life. The dismissal of my empirical based summary paper, by equivocating it with "contrary opinions available on the Internet" brought me to tears. Angry, rage-filled, tears. But I had little recourse. They were the medical assessor, paid by Immigration New Zealand, to consider my medical reports and make an assessment on whether I met the standard of acceptable health. Because of my BMI, I did not.

Round 4

I didn't meet the acceptable standard of health. Therefore, to gain a visa, I would need to apply for a medical waiver. A medical waiver would be granted after the immigration officers considered the circumstances of my application and whether there was compelling enough evidence to justify me being allowed to stay and work in New Zealand, even without meeting the acceptable standard of health. To facilitate this process, I hired the best immigration lawyer in the country. Luckily, I had the personal connections to get me in the door of the firm and the financial resources to pay for their services.

The case made by the lawyer was twofold. First, that it was wrong of the medical assessors to suggest that I would impose costs or demands on New Zealand's health system. He noted that all three assessors ticked the box referring to "chronic recurring medical condition," yet I had none. He also drew attention that, "Two of the medical assessors refer to no evidentiary basis for their views; and the third refers to certain generalised instead." And he noted that the opinions show the assessors have been addressing costs which I *could* or *might* impose, not what I *would* impose. He argued that the assessors failed to prove I *would* impose costs or demands on the health system of New Zealand.

The second point was that I had demonstrated, through my own statement and statements provided by five witnesses, that my potential contribution to New Zealand would be significant. Statement writers included the vice-chancellor of my university, the pro vice-chancellor of my college, three academics from Australasia, and my local member of parliament. These letters all emphasized the contributions I had made to New Zealand in my three years of work thus far, and the future contributions I was sure to make if allowed to remain.

Unfortunately, in the closing of his statement, my lawyer drew upon the good fatty archetype to support his argument that I should be granted a medical waiver. There are many good fatty archetypes (see the work of Bias 2014), with the unifying theme being the performance or embodiment of fatness that is most palatable to our fat-hating society (Pausé 2015); for example, a fat person who talks openly about their attempts at weight loss, or always order the salad in a restaurant. Other good fatty performances may include insisting on being in good health, despite or while being fat. As noted, my lawyer made two points in his brief: that the assessors did not establish that I *would* impose costs or demands on the health system, and that my potential contribution to New Zealand would be significant enough to outweigh any possible costs or demands regardless. In his closing, he stressed, "We emphasize that Dr. Pausé's situation is unique in that she does not have health conditions. Dr. Pausé should be granted a health waiver."

And my lawyer wasn't the only one who drew on the good fatty to support his arguments. In the penultimate paragraph of the letter of support from my pro vice-chancellor, he noted that in the three years I had been in his faculty, "there have been no health issues that have in any way impeded her from performing her academic duties." While I appreciate that this was said to directly challenge the suggestion that my weight might impede my ability to work made by the initial medical assessment (as drafted by Assessor 1), I found it cringeworthy then and I find it cringe worthy now. Real damage is done by reinforcing the idea that if I had health issues (related to my weight or not) that had impeded me from performing my job I would be less worthy of my job, or a residency visa, or my humanity. But I can also recognize that I used the good fatty archetype myself in my attempt to obtain my visa. I specifically told the endocrinologist, without being prompted, that I ate healthily and regularly exercised; I'm sure I played this up to all of the healthcare professionals I saw during this process.

The aftermath

In the end, I was awarded a medical waiver and granted a resident visa. But the process was extremely stressful. It spanned almost an entire year, encompassing repeated trips to have blood drawn, and repeated short-term visa applications to allow me to stay in the country while my case was being decided. I felt frozen; unable to plan and continue building the life in New Zealand I desired, but unwilling to accept defeat and begin planning a very different future for myself. I was depressed, anxious, mad as hell at the situation, and embarrassed as well.

Consider that this was my experience, as a person with a great deal of privilege. I'm a white, cis, straight, well-educated person from the United States of America. I held a well-paying job that allowed for the financial resources to pay for temporary work permits, medical expenses, specialist visits, and, eventually, a lawyer. In addition, my job as a member of the professoriate bestows an amount of prestige and esteem that helped me procure letters of support from well-respected members of my community in positions of power. I was also lucky to have the support of my family, friends, and colleagues during the ordeal. None of them being "super" fat, they lacked an understanding of the nuance of the situation or the cognitive dissonance that arises when what I know and believe (that's it is not okay to deny someone humanity based on their size) clashes with what I've internalized my entire life (that my fatness is my fault and it is bad and I deserve all the bad things that come from it). And many, while trying to be supportive, actually played into the same ideas that my humanity was somehow connected to my health status or ability to produce labor. For example, a close colleague in human resources at my university suggested that a work around might be if I were to promise or agree to purchase and hold private health insurance, to alleviate concerns of the cost to the public system. He failed to see that this would make me a second-class citizen, denied to entitlements granted to everyone else, based on my weight. Solovay (2000) suggested that fat stigma and discrimination have resulted in fat people living as second-class citizens already.

It was stressful, alienating, and isolating.[1] But in the end, I was awarded residency (which then led to permanent residency and citizenship). Others, like Albert Buitenhuis, have not been so lucky. He worked in New Zealand for years on temporary work visas, and was never able to secure something more permanent (Miller 2015); there are many others as well (Fox News 2007; Piddington 2009). For me, my BMI alone, and the predictions they linked to my BMI, allowed them to conclude that I did not meet the acceptable standard of health to be granted residency in New Zealand. And New Zealand isn't alone in this tactic; many other Western countries employ similar procedures, such as Australia, the United States, and the United Kingdom. Firth (2012) argued that "citizenship provides a framework in which neoliberalism, biopolitics, and the 'obesity epidemic' can be brought together" (40); a perfect storm, as it were. I've shared my experience with navigating the process of immigration as a super fat person to illuminate how state structures (re)produce fat oppression. In this system, fat bodies "are failures. They are the abnormal that delineates the boundary of normalcy. In this way, fat bodies quite helpfully delineate the boundaries between good and bad citizenship" (Owen 2015, 5). Fat activists and others working to progress social justice must expand their efforts to include barriers set by countries that limit the ability of fat people to live and work where they please. As noted by Murray (2005), I can't love myself to citizenship. These structural oppressions have to be addressed as civil rights issues, so people of all sizes may have the liberty to live where they please.

Note

1. And this has been true for completing this work as well. Never before have I experienced such discomfort in conducting a piece of scholarship. While I have completed other autoethnographic pieces of work, this one impacted me in a way I hadn't fully expected. I did expect the feelings of shame and anger and despair and frustration to arise as I delved into the "Immigration" file I constructed over the year's battle. I wasn't prepared, however, for how much I had to battle to keep those feelings from completely overwhelming me as I constructed this piece.

References

Bacchi, C. L., and C. Beasley. 2002. "Citizen Bodies: Is Embodied Citizenship a Contradiction in Terms?" *Critical Social Policy* 22 (2):324–52. doi: 10.1177/02610183020220020801.

Bias, S. 2014. "12 Good Fatty Archetypes." Stacy Bias [Web blog post]. Accessed June 4. http://stacybias.net/2014/06/12-good-fatty-archetypes/.

Blank, H.. n.d "Letter to a Doctor." Cat and Dragon [Web blog post]. http://cat-and-dragon.com/stef/fat/hanne.html.

Brackenridge, R. D. C. 1985. *Medical Selection of Life Risks: A Comprehensive Guide to Life Expectancy for Underwriters & Clinicians*. 2nd ed. London: Nature Press.

Byers, M. 2018. ""Fats," Futurity, and the Contemporary Young Adult Novel." *Fat Studies* 7 (2):159–69. doi:10.1080/21604851.2017.1373242.

Campos, P., A. Saguy, P. Ernsberger, E. Oliver, and G. Gaesser. 2005. "The Epidemiology of Overweight and Obesity: Public Health Crisis or Moral Panic?" *International Journal of Epidemiology* 35 (1):55–60. doi:10.1093/ije/dyi254.

Cooper, C. 2016. *Fat Activism: A Radical Social Movement*. Bristol, England: HammerOn Press.

Elliott, C. D. 2007. "Big Persons, Small Voices: On Governance, Obesity, and the Narrative of the Failed Citizen." *Journal of Canadian Studies* 41 (3):134–49. doi:10.3138/jcs.41.3.134.

Ellis, C., T. E. Adams, and A. P. Bochner. 2011. "Autoethnography: An Overview." *Historical Social Research/Historische Sozialforschung* 36 (4):273–90.

Firth, J. 2012. "Healthy Choices and Heavy Burdens: Race, Citizenship and Gender in the 'Obesity Epidemic'." *Journal of International Women's Studies* 13 (2):33.

Foster, G. D., T. A. Wadden, A. P. Makris, D. Davidson, R. S. Sanderson, D. B. Allison, and A. Kessler. 2003. "Primary Care Physicians' Attitudes about Obesity and Its Treatment." *Obesity* 11 (10):1168–77. doi:10.1038/oby.2003.161.

Foucault, M. 1990. *The History of Sexuality, Vol 1: The Will to Knowledge*. London: Penguin.

Fox News. 2007. "New Zealand Denies Immigration to U.K. Wife because She's Too Fat. Fox News, Reposting from the Daily Mail [Online Edition]." Accessed November 17. http://www.foxnews.com/story/2007/11/17/new-zealand-denies-immigration-to-uk-wife-because-too-fat.html.

Fox, R. 2018. "Against Progress: Understanding and Resisting the Temporality of Transformational Weight Loss Narratives." *Fat Studies* 7 (2):216–26. doi:10.1080/21604851.2017.1372992.

Harjunen, H. 2016. *Neoliberal Bodies and the Gendered Fat Body*. London, UK: Routledge.

Hass, M. 2018. "One Summer to Change: Fat Temporality and Coming of Age in I Used to Be Fat and Huge." *Fat Studies* 170–81. doi: 10.1080/21604851.2017.1372991.

Hebl, M. R., and J. Xu. 2001. "Weighing the Care: Physicians' Reactions to the Size of a Patient." *International Journal of Obesity* 25 (8):1246. doi:10.1038/sj.ijo.0801742.

Herndon, A. 2005. "Collateral Damage from Friendly Fire? Race, Nation, Class, and the "War against Obesity"." *Social Semiotics* 15 (2):127–41. doi:10.1080/10350330500154634.

Immigration New Zealand. 2016. General Medical Certificate. Ministry of Business, Innovation & Employment. Accessed November. https://www.immigration.govt.nz/documents/forms-and-guides/inz1007.pdf.

Immigration New Zealand. "Health." https://www.immigration.govt.nz/new-zealand-visas/apply-for-a-visa/about-visa/talent-accredited-employers-work-to-residence-visa#https://www.immigration.govt.nz/new-zealand-visas/apply-for-a-visa/tools-and-information/general-information/travelling-to-and-arriving-in-new-zealand/slider.

Immigration New Zealand. "Welcome." https://www.immigration.govt.nz/new-zealand-visas.

Jutel, A. 2006. "The Emergence of Overweight as a Disease Entity: Measuring up Normality." *Social Science & Medicine* 63 (9):2268–76. doi:10.1016/j.socscimed.2006.05.028.

LeBesco, K. 2011. "Neoliberalism, Public Health, and the Moral Perils of Fatness." *Critical Public Health* 21 (2):153–64. doi:10.1080/09581596.2010.529422.

Lee, J. A., and C. J. Pausé. 2016. "Stigma in Practice: Barriers to Health for Fat Women." *Frontiers in Psychology* 7:2063. doi: 10.3389/fpsyg.2016.02063.

Miller, C. 2015. "'Too Fat' Chef Gives up Immigration Battle, Wants NZ to Send Him His Cat. New Zealand Herald [Online Edition]." Accessed December 18. http://www.nzherald.co.nz/nz/news/article.cfm?c_id=1&objectid=11563096.

Murray, S. 2005. "(Un/Be) Coming Out? Rethinking Fat Politics." *Social Semiotics* 15 (2):153–63. doi:10.1080/10350330500154667.

Owen, L. J. 2015. "Monstrous Freedom: Charting Fat Ambivalence." *Fat Studies* 4 (1):1–13. doi:10.1080/21604851.2014.896186.

Pace, G. 2006. "Obesity Bigger Threat than Terrorism?" CBS News. Accessed March 1. https://www.cbsnews.com/news/obesity-bigger-threat-than-terrorism.

Parker, G., and C. J. Pausé. 2018. "Pregnant with Possibility: Negotiating Fat Maternal Subjectivity in the "War on Obesity"." *Fat Studies: an Interdisciplinary Journal of Body Weight & Society* 7 (2):124–34. doi:10.1080/21604851.2017.1372990.

Pausé, C. 2012a. "Live to Tell: Coming Out as Fat." *Somatechnics* 2 (1):42–56. doi:10.3366/soma.2012.0038.

Pausé, C. 2012b. "On the Epistemology of Fatness." Friend of Marilyn [Web blog post]. Accessed April 5. https://friendofmarilyn.com/2012/04/05/the-epistemology-of-fatness/.

Pausé, C. J. 2014. "Die Another Day: The Obstacles Facing Fat People in Accessing Shame-Free and Evidenced-Based Healthcare." *Narrative Inquiry in Bioethics* 4 (3):135–41. doi:10.1353/nib.2014.0039.

Pausé, C. J. 2015. "Rebel Heart: Performing Fatness Wrong Online." *M/C Journal* 18 (3). Retrieved from http://journal.media-culture.org.au/index.php/mcjournal/article/viewArticle/977.

Piddington, S. 2009. "Doctor Too Big for NZ. Timaru Herald [Online edition, Stuff]." Accessed May 11, http://www.stuff.co.nz/timaru-herald/news/2376954/Doctor-too-big-for-NZ.

Pollack, A. 2013. "A.M.A. Recognises Obesity as a Disease." *New York Times* [Online edition]. Accessed June 18. https://www.nytimes.com/2013/06/19/business/ama-recognizes-obesity-as-a-disease.html.

Prospective Studies Collaboration. 2009. "Body-Mass Index and Cause-Specific Mortality in 900 000 Adults: Collaborative Analyses of 57 Prospective Studies." *The Lancet* 373 (9669):1083–96. doi: 10.1016/S0140-6736(09)60318-4.

Rinaldi, J., C. Rice, A. LaMarre, D. McPhail, and E. Harrison. 2017. "Fatness and Failing Citizenship." *Somatechnics* 7 (2):218–33. doi:10.3366/soma.2017.0219.

Solovay, S. 2000. *Tipping the Scales of Justice*. Amherst, New York, USA: Prometheus Books.

Swinburn, B., T. Ashton, J. Gillespie, B. Cox, A. Menon, D. Simmons, and J. Birbeck. 1997. "Health Care Costs of Obesity in New Zealand." *International Journal of Obesity* 21:891–96.

Can ambivalence hold potential for fat activism? An analysis of conflicting discourses on fatness in the Finnish column series *Jenny's Life Change*

Anna Puhakka

ABSTRACT

In 2017, a publicly funded, nationwide campaign called the Scale Rebellion set out to address fatness through body positivity and fat activism in Finland, with a fat woman named Jenny Lehtinen having a particularly visible role as its figurehead. Some critics of the campaign maintained that Lehtinen's communication lacked focus and was self-contradicting, especially concerning her wish to lose weight. I conducted discourse analysis of a pertinent element of the Scale Rebellion campaign, a 13-part column series called *Jenny's Life Change*, written by Lehtinen herself. The findings suggest that diverse, conflicting discourses on fatness are indeed present in her texts; of these, I have named anti-"obesity," fatphobic, size acceptance, and societal discourses. However, in line with scholars such as Michalinos Zembylas, I argue that Lehtinen's conflicting messaging on fatness is not (only) an expression of her personal opinions but in fact linked to ambivalent fatness discourses circulating in Finnish society and abroad. Further, Samantha Murray has noted that fat activism would do well in welcoming the multivocality often present in (narratives on) fatness, since ambivalence might actually contain potential. One such possibility is the very observation that ambivalence vis-à-vis fatness is not necessarily a sign of being a sell-out or a "fake" fat activist. Instead, it is an indication that at a time when fatness is a stigmatized trait, almost everyone is exposed to conflicting messages about it. Therefore fat activists' ambivalence in relation to fatness should not be judged but rather seen in this larger context.

Introduction

"… fat activism does not have to be coherent in order to be valid." (Cooper 2016, 92)

Like many other countries, Finnish society—the media included—is saturated with one-sided accounts of fat: how it destroys (public) health and how to best get rid of it. A dramatic change came in 2017: The country's public service broadcasting company, Yle, launched a year-long, multichannel (Internet, TV, and radio) body positivity campaign called the Scale Rebellion (*Vaakakapina*), with "Stop Dieting, Start Living" as its slogan. Finns followed journalist Jenny Lehtinen, the campaign's figurehead and a self-proclaimed fat woman, in her quest for a renewed relationship with her body through columns, TV appearances, and intense social media. Two weeks after the Scale Rebellion ended, Yle called it the "people's movement that put an end to crash diets" (Yle 2018).

Not everyone was impressed, however. Critics grew frustrated with the Scale Rebellion because they were unable to figure out its final message: In the end, did it advise the public to lose weight or not (E. Soikkeli, personal communication, March 15, 2018)? In particular, Jenny Lehtinen's ambivalence toward her own fatness was highlighted. The credibility of the campaign was seen to be compromised because its body positive leader ostensibly couldn't make up her mind about whether she herself wanted to be thin or not (Juti 2017). Her columns, written in a personal—and at times emotional—tone, were perceived to reflect these conflicting feelings.

Nevertheless, in this article, I attempt a different reading of this ambivalence. In line with scholars such as Zembylas (2012), I propose that interpreting the *Jenny's Life Change* (*Jennyn elämänmuutos*) columns—part of the Scale Rebellion campaign—that provide the data for this article as if they were solely private musings, and focusing on the columnist as an individual (as some of the critics have done), might not be very productive. Instead, it is more fruitful to examine how her writing might reflect the diverse fatness discourses circulating in contemporary Finnish society (as well as abroad, given the easy access to information produced elsewhere). When the focus is shifted from Lehtinen's conflicting messaging on fatness as an expression of her personal opinions to how the different discourses evoked in the columns are linked to ambivalent discourses moving about in society, it becomes easier to discern how they often conflict each other and are thus more likely to lead to very different understandings of a phenomenon—fatness, in this case.

What is more, Samantha Murray, among others, has suggested that the ambivalence often felt vis-à-vis fat embodiment may contain potential, particularly in the context of fat politics (Murray 2005, 2008, 2010). I offer that one such possibility is the realization that at a time when fatness is a stigmatized trait, ambivalence points to the fact that almost everyone is exposed to conflicting messages about it. This includes those who are supposed to fight against this stigma—such as body positivity and fat activists (Ayuso 2001; Cooper 1998, 2016; Donaghue and Clemitshaw 2012; Maor 2013b; McMichael 2010; Meleo-Erwin 2011; Murray 2005, 2008, 2010). Put differently, given the extent of these various discourses, experienced ambiguity toward fatness is not necessarily a sign of being a sell-out or a "fake" fat activist. Therefore, activists' ambivalence toward fatness should not be judged—as some critics of the Scale Rebellion have done—but rather seen in this larger context.

This article is, to my knowledge, the first to examine the Scale Rebellion, as it is very recent. In addition, Finnish fat activism deserves to be documented and analyzed so that the now-existing supply of information on fat activism "can be made known, archived, made into further resources for people to adopt" (Cooper and Murray 2012, 134, in Maor 2013a, 281). Moreover, the present study answers the call to geographically and culturally diversify fat studies (Cooper 2009; see also Maor 2013a). This is important since "fat rights initiatives outside the United States ... at worst, are exoticized, belittled, or unnoticed" (Cooper 2009, 330).

Fat activism, ambivalence, and discourse

The starting point of this study is that fat activism is a valid form of resilience in the face of fat oppression. Fat activism has been characterized as "a social movement concerned with fatness that has many sites and interests" (Cooper 2016, 2). But because the Scale Rebellion calls itself "the biggest *body positivity* revolution in Finland" (Scale Rebellion n.d.; emphasis mine) on its home page, I want to address why I deem it appropriate to consider the campaign as expressly fat activism. It seems to me that this choice of vocabulary has been made at least partly because "as a concept," "body positivity" is more familiar to Finns than "fat activism"—in other words, the former sounds more palatable than the latter. This doesn't mean, however, that the Scale Rebellion is not fat activism.

In her book, *Fat Activism*, Charlotte Cooper argues that "fat activism covers a range of interventions and ... many different activities can be thought of as activism" (Cooper 2016, 93). She points out that as many other forms of activism, fat activism, too, can even be contradictory, in opposition to what has traditionally been thought. Further, Cooper calls some forms of fat activism "ambiguous" and asserts that they emerge when produced "by people who are 'failed' or 'less-than-ideal' fat activists" (Cooper 2016, 88).

Interestingly, it is precisely ambiguous fat activism that is characterized by puzzlement over the fact that "its context, execution and effects [are] not very straightforward" (Cooper 2016, 85). Moreover, Cooper describes this type of activism thus: "[It] can be provocative and it upsets notions of propriety, purpose and progression in activism" (Cooper 2016, 87). This echoes the Finnish public's mixed reactions concerning the Scale Rebellion: The campaign has stirred up lively discussions, online and off. Accordingly then, that the Scale Rebellion perhaps does not follow long-established ways of doing activism does not mean it is not activism—it just may be characterized by ambivalence.

Although admittedly an everyday occurrence (Preckel et al. 2015), ambivalence is rarely perceived as a strength; ambivalence regarding fatness specifically has often been portrayed as a negative phenomenon. When one grows up in a culture that clearly favors a particular body type above all others, those not fitting in will at times feel conflicted about their different embodiment, no matter how immersed in activism (Pausé 2017). In recent years, numerous studies have been conducted where fatness and ambivalence have featured prominently (Gruys 2012; Hardin 2015; Kyrölä and Harjunen 2017; White 2014). Still others have discussed ambivalence particularly in the context of fat activism or fat politics— concepts I will use interchangeably (Cooper 1998; Donaghue and Clemitshaw 2012; LeBesco 2004; Maor 2013a; McMichael 2010; Meleo-Erwin 2011, 2012). It appears that ambivalence in relation to fatness is far from a rare occurrence. Nevertheless, not many of these contributions make allusion to the *potential* of ambivalence in fat activism.

In her 2005 article, "(Un/Be)Coming Out? Rethinking Fat Politics," Samantha Murray's focus is on fat politics and its (assumed; cf. Cooper 2016, 14–18) demand for "a fat subject with a stable and unitary 'resisting' consciousness … that univocally rejects dominant views of fat and is able to fully accept her or his body" (Maor 2013a, 281). Coming from a phenomenological stance, Murray points to the ever-changing nature of the human experience and the impossibility of capturing it in a single still frame. She urges us to acknowledge the constant, internal tug of war a fat woman is faced with: On one hand, there is the call for loving one's body unconditionally, and on the other, the negative discourses that cannot *not* influence the way that body is perceived and experienced.

Murray argues that we "cannot experience our bodies in singular, unambiguous ways. This reality, then, needs to be accommodated in ways where ambivalence does not have to be a kind of guilty secret, but is productive in terms of opening out multiple ways of being" (Murray 2008, 144). Maya Maor (2013b) has subsequently reemphasized the potential for resistance and change that fatness's ambivalence carries, as has Owen (2015). In Samantha Murray's words: "If 'coming out' as fat refuses an ambiguous identity, then it refuses *the possibilities ambiguity presents*" (Murray 2005, 62; emphasis mine).

Zembylas's work (2012) on ambivalent discourses is of interest here. Zembylas interviewed Greek-Cypriot children and youth, concentrating on the descriptions of their feelings about migrants in Cyprus. He found not only that these portrayals were complex and conflicted but, even more importantly, that the interviewees' "emotions [were] linked to ambivalent discourses," themselves framed in the societal level (Zembylas 2012, 195).

Zembylas underscores that the main point of his article is not whether his study participants' perceptions were negative or positive. Instead, his study's contribution is that "overall these participants have perceptions of migrants that are fed by ambivalent emotion discourses" (Zembylas 2012, 205). One of the possibilities ambivalence presents for fat activism, then, resides in the fact that once we realize that ambiguity is not an individual-level phenomenon (at least, not solely)—for instance, Jenny Lehtinen's columns are *not* about one woman who is unable to make up her mind about dieting—the door is opened for us to turn our gaze toward the wider circumstance of discourse.

According to a seminal work on discourse analysis, rather than defining it as a "research method with clear-cut boundaries, it is more meaningful to think of discourse analysis as *a loose theoretical framework*" (Jokinen, Juhila, and Suoninen 1993, 17; emphasis in original). This useful approach has helped me not only to discern between different discourses but also to analyze them in more depth.

The Finnish context

The negative attributes attached to fat persons, familiar from other parts of the world—lazy, dirty, stupid, and ugly (Rissanen and Mustajoki 2006, 120)—prevail in Finland as well (Mustajoki 2018). Fat people are discriminated against in employment (Härkönen and Räsänen 2008; Kauppinen and Anttila 2005) and social life (Rissanen and Mustajoki 2006), among others.

Consequently, antifat attitudes have found their way into several cultural products. Among the most prominent are international weight-loss TV formats such as *The Biggest Loser*, as well as their domestic counterparts, like *Honey, You've Become Chubby* (*Rakas, sinusta on tullut pullukka*, aired in 2013-2016) and *Jutta's Six-Month Superdiets* (*Jutta ja puolen vuoden super-dieetit*, aired in 2013-2015). Many magazines boast a regular weight-loss section, and the Internet is full of diverse service providers, coaches, nutritionists, and personal trainers aiming to help Finns become thin. Not surprisingly in this overall context, in 2016, only 16 percent of women and 22 percent of men in Finland were happy with their weight (Yle 2017).

Finally, when discussing different discourses circulating in Finnish society, it is important to look beyond those produced in Finnish and Swedish, the official languages of the country. For instance, ten years ago, 82 percent of Finnish adults aged 18-64 said they knew English at least somewhat (Statistics Finland 2008). This enables the acquisition of information from other linguistic regions, such as the anglophone United States, Great Britain, and Australia, where alarmist discourses about fatness have been active for a long period of time—as has counter speech (see, e.g., Cooper 2010). Further, this information acquisition is greatly facilitated by an almost unconstrained access to the Internet (Statistics Finland 2017). In other words, Finns' access to different discourses is high.

Overview of the case study and methodology

As noted, the Scale Rebellion was a year-long multichannel media campaign taking place in 2017. Its central themes were summarized in the *Scale Rebellion Manifesto*: stop dieting; find love and acceptance for the body; improve the way fatness is approached in the health-care system; bring forth bodies of all sizes in the media, without expressing outrage; and make exercise and health-care services genuinely accessible for everyone (Yle 2018).

The Finnish Broadcasting Company, Yle, who produced the Scale Rebellion, is a public service company. As such, it is 99.98 percent owned by the Finnish state—or actually Finns, because a special Yle tax has been in place since 2013 (Yle n.d.). This fact spurred a municipal politician to rhetorically ask whether the campaign's purpose was to rebel against scales or to show strong opposition against "common sense and public health, with the taxpayers' money" instead (Hyttinen 2017).

The Scale Rebellion has stirred up other online discussions as well. More often than not, when critique has been presented, it has been aimed at the overall campaign. Instead of focusing on specific components, many contributors have questioned the campaign's raison d'être. A participant in a now-archived Reddit thread comments: "Fatlogic keeps on spreading... . America is leading and Finland is not far behind" (Anonymous n.d.), while a local newspaper columnist writes: "The rise in obesity has come to a halt [in Finland], but not because people have gotten happy with their weight and bodies" (Tahvanainen 2017). On the other hand, there are bloggers who support the campaign, pointing out, for example, that it is promoting human rights (Sieluni silmin 2018) and meant for everyone, no matter the size (Ylönen 2017).

A 13-part column series, *Jenny's Life Change*, a pertinent part of the Scale Rebellion, constitutes the data for this article (Lehtinen n.d.). The online series was spread across the year, with a column appearing approximately once a month. The topics match those of the *Scale Rebellion Manifesto*; some monthly themes, such as health care, were discussed in conjunction with other components, such as video clips. The average length of the columns was 607 words, but there was considerable variation: The shortest text contained 342 words, while the longest comprised 1128 words.[1]

To analyze the data, I used qualitative content analysis, since it "focuses on the characteristics of language as communication with attention to the content or contextual meaning of the text" (Hsieh and Shannon 2005, 1278). In other words, qualitative content analysis is not (only) concerned with counting occurrences; rather, it aims to probe into the meaning of the words, subsequently grouping them by shared similarities. After particular themes—discourses—started to emerge from the data, I applied purposeful sampling to select the extracts that illustrated the phenomenon under discussion in the most information-rich manner (Palinkas et al. 2015).

This particular group of texts was chosen because they were written by the campaign leader Jenny Lehtinen. I assume that function allowed her the leeway to express herself without limit or restraint. This is valuable, given that this study's purpose is to investigate conflicting discourses in the texts.

Findings and discussion

With discourse analysis as my main interpretative tool, I distinguished four main discourses in the data: anti-"obesity," fatphobic, size acceptance, and societal.

Anti-"obesity" discourse

To characterize the first thematic set of texts, I am using Deborah Lupton's (2018) term anti-"obesity" discourse. Additional terms often synonymous to it are "obesity discourse" (e.g., Monaghan, Colls, and Evans 2013), and "obesity epidemic discourse" (see Harjunen 2017). I chose Lupton's terminology because firstly and most obviously, "obesity" figures in it, indicating that this discourse sees fatness as "a disease or a precursor to disease" (Lupton 2018, 26). What is more, the prefix *anti-* makes it clear that "obesity" is something to be eradicated.

> Being overweight and having body image issues are not a failure due to a person's weaknesses, but caused by a sum of various individual, cultural, and social factors. And when that's recognized and acknowledged, folks can really get help with their problems. (#2)[2]

In this section, Jenny Lehtinen does emphasize that "being overweight" does not equal lack of success, clearly aware that this is the prevailing stereotype (Jutel 2005; Puhl et al. 2015; Solovay and Rothblum 2009). At the same time, she can be seen to perpetuate the frequently held assumption that fatness is rooted in individual pathology, such as mental illness (Orbach 1978; for an extensive summary, see Cooper 2010). Moreover, she seems to have adopted the notion, common in medicine and public health, that in the end, fatness is a hurdle: She alludes to "overweight" and body image issues collectively as "problems." Another excerpt, later in the same column, lends this interpretation of fatness-as-problem further credence:

> And does it make sense to tell a person to lose weight if they're healthy but weigh too much? Can we leave them alone as long as relevant indicators, such as blood tests, are OK, even though their BMI wouldn't fit within the ideal? (#2)

Similarly, this excerpt contains manifest elements typical of the anti-"obesity" discourse. First, the wording "weigh too much" betrays the columnist's view that there *is* such a thing as weighing too much. This echoes Western medicine with its firm emphasis on quantification, measuring, BMI charts, and overall normativization (Lupton 2018). Second, a strong undercurrent of healthism is present when the writer claims that it's accep-table to be fat "as long as relevant indicators ... are OK." This viewpoint has been criticized with vehemence. Using the figures of the good fatty and the bad fatty, commentators have pointed out that this logic divides fat people into two camps (Pausé 2015; Rose Water Magazine 2015). The good fatties are those who eat a wholesome diet and exercise regularly. The bad fatties, in turn, are constructed as ignorant sloths who have only themselves to blame if and when they get sick. The neoliberal logic of free will and individual choice further feeds into this rationalization (Harjunen 2017; Lupton 2018).

Fatphobic discourse

While fatphobia is certainly not an unknown phenomenon in Finnish society, it was still surprising to find outright fatphobic discourse in the columns. Although nearly everyone in Finland is at one point or another exposed to the fear of fatness and fat people, it still felt out of place to see fatphobia in the context of an explicitly body positive campaign, created by media professionals, and with nationwide coverage. Nonetheless, I don't think this translates as Jenny Lehtinen being a particularly fatphobic indivi-dual; the juxtaposition of these elements provides a startling example of ambivalence.

> Oftentimes, people measure or want to measure my "success" by whether I have lost weight.... . It's also something people speculate on, and sometimes even ask me to my face: does Jenny Lehtinen want to lose weight? I do. I want my weight to become normalized. In my wildest (and pretty sick) fantasies, often still thumping in the back of my head, I would like to lose half of my body weight. And even if I say that I never ever want to lose weight again, that's a lie as well. I do want to lose weight, every single day, many times. (#11)

The writer is very open about her wanting to diet and her wish to lose a drastic amount of weight. Fat activists and celebrities (as a media person, Jenny Lehtinen is quite a visible figure) are not immune to this kind of ambivalence. *Fat Heffalump* blogger Kath Read, for instance, has written about internalized fatphobia and the responsibility of prominent fat persons to consider the consequences to fat people in general when the former decide to lose weight (Read 2017). She asserts that, in fact, famous ex-fat folks end up reinforcing the existing narratives, in other words strengthening the piece of conventional wisdom that being fat is simply not desirable. Writing about three categories of public figures' positions in relation to their own fatness, Kathleen LeBesco discusses what she calls Traitors. They are those who, when fat, talk openly about feeling good in their bodies and not wanting to change, only to turn to dieting or weight-loss surgery later on, giving an utterly hypocritical impression of themselves (LeBesco 2004, 92–97).

Still, after all [the fat activism], I caught myself recently passing on fatphobia to my child. When they asked me … if I thought they were fat, I was quick to reply: "Oh no, of course not! Goodness! Absolutely not!" … I realized that the way I handled my child's question contained a hidden message: It would be just awful if you were fat. … And above all, I should understand and accept this idea myself: my body is precious and beloved exactly as it is. (#6)

It is obvious that the columnist is aware of, first, that the ubiquitous fatphobic discourse exists, and second, that she has been affected by it—otherwise it would be impossible to pass on fatphobia to her own child. Charlotte Cooper has noted that despite all their work against fat bias, fat activists sometimes "still end up back at square one, blaming [their] bodies for [their] oppression and feeling overwhelmed by [their] fatness" (Cooper 1998, 57–58).

Size acceptance discourse

A third discourse distinguishable from the columns is what I have termed size acceptance discourse. It comes close to body positivity (notably, a form of fat activism itself; Cooper 2016) in that unconditional love for one's body is an integral part of it:

> You can and are allowed to love your body, no matter what it's like. The only thing the kilograms can define about you is what the body weighs. (#2)

Body positive fat activist Marilyn Wann, for example, has exhorted her readers to "Ask yourself, what has body anxiety done for me lately? Nothing good, right? So why not get rid of it??? … You just have to change your attitude" (Wann 1998, 13). Here the possibility of fully accepting one's body through changing one's mind (cf. Murray 2005, 2008, 2010) is palpably present. But Jenny Lehtinen expresses caution with regard to this attitudinal transformation:

> Many have written [at a related Facebook group] about how difficult it feels to actually genuinely accept oneself. That even if you're all for the idea, it's still empty words and repetition without real content. Hey, we're all in the same boat! This is how it is in the beginning. If certain structures have built up in your mind for years and decades, it takes time to change them. For some, it takes longer, for others, less. I'm one of the former. (#8)

This quote demonstrates that the columnist is cognizant of the ambivalent discourses that make it difficult to adhere to body positive fat activists' calls for unconditional self-acceptance. In an interview, Hannele Harjunen has remarked that the point of departure for size acceptance in general, and for the Scale Rebellion in particular, is problematic in that the responsibility for change is bestowed upon the individual (Laapotti 2017, 19). According to Charlotte Cooper, size acceptance has "a resigned feel to it" (Cooper 2008, n. p.); fat liberation ideas have been diluted when introduced to mainstream culture and becoming connected to the fashion and beauty industries, in turn producing "a more tentative approach to fat" (Cooper 2008, n.p.).

Societal discourse

I have chosen to name this discourse "societal" because instead of focusing on the individual, as body positivity discourse can be seen to do (cf. Omaheimo and Särmä 2017), societal discourse takes a bird's eye view, looking at "human beings thought of as a group and viewed as members of a community" ("Society" n.d.):

> The Scale Rebellion is about people ... questioning the status quo as regards what kind of a body is good enough, and might [their bodies] be like that. And really find the best way for them to live.... . A good life is dependent on so many factors, certainly not on body size only. (#11)

Lehtinen urges her readers to challenge the current situation and societal norms, and this is not the first time. In 2016, before starting the Scale Rebellion, Jenny Lehtinen was a reporter in another Yle television show, *Marja Hintikka Live*. A regular segment of the program was *Jenny and the FatMythBusters* (alluding to the popular TV series MythBusters), whose themes were similar to the Scale Rebellion. Possibly the most significant outcome of the FatMythBusters was its Facebook group which continues to be active to this day. In June 2018, it had 31,720 members (of all sizes), and there are several posts every day: link shares, photos, and personal stories. Conceivably propelled by this success, the Scale Rebellion was launched, and it is evident that Lehtinen's columns do speak to many of the anxieties voiced in the FatMythBusters Facebook group:

> I want to give people back the right to their own bodies: You are not ugly. Not worthless. You are not a walking health risk. You are a human being with the right to define your body exactly the way you want to. You are allowed to be healthy, beautiful, athletic, hard working, sexy, whatever you want. You also have the right to be treated with dignity everywhere, no matter what you weigh. (#2)

Although Lehtinen's writing style is very vocal, she is not the first media personality to publicly interrogate fat oppression in Finland. One of the first avenues to confront antifat attitudes was the blog *More to Love*. It was active during 2009–2013 and wanted to "represent all the big and beautiful ladies in Finland" (More to Love n.d.). Discussion on Finnish intersectional fat activism is said to have properly begun only in 2016 (Omaheimo and Särmä 2017). It is from then on that activists have started to openly question widespread antifat bias in the form of numerous blogs (such as Vatsamielenosoitus n.d.), Internet sites (e.g., Merimaa and Stolt n.d.), and a theater monologue "Fatso" (*"Läski"*; Omaheimo and Kilkku 2016).

It is noteworthy that multiple—even seemingly contradicting—discourses are emergent within a single column at times. One example is article #2, where anti-"obesity," size acceptance, and societal discourses are all present. Another instance is article #11, which contains elements of both fatphobic and societal discourses. This demonstrates that instead of Jenny Lehtinen merely referencing the disagreeing opinions on fatness in the society, she is holding inconsistent and even contradictory beliefs and feelings about fatness herself. Furthermore, there is considerable interaction between the discourses. While they have been presented here as distinct for reasons of clarity, in reality, they are simultaneously intertwined.

Conclusions

The Scale Rebellion was an extensive campaign with a broad coverage; as such, it took the public discussion on fatness to a new level in Finland. In many ways, the campaign came to equal the outspoken Jenny Lehtinen. But although the texts analyzed are written by a particular individual, this study's point is not to draw attention on Lehtinen specifically. Neither is my intention to label the discourses discernible in the columns simply "good" or "bad." Instead, inspired by Zembylas's work, it seems that a more productive approach could be looking at how the different discourses evoked in the analyzed texts are linked to ambivalent discourses circulating in contemporary Finnish society and elsewhere (Zembylas 2012, 195; see also Murray 2010).

According to my analysis, fatness is a phenomenon that, in the *Jenny's Life Change* columns at least, is currently discussed through discourses that I have named anti-"obesity," fatphobic, size acceptance, and societal. As a columnist, Jenny Lehtinen has had access to and been influenced by all of these different discourses—among many others, undoubtedly. They have shaped how she, in turn, is presenting fatness in her own work.

This is why it is problematic to interpret Lehtinen's writing as a mere reflection of her personal inability to make up her mind about being fat. Ignoring the role of discourses and calling fat activists—as Jenny Lehtinen was by a critic—"'a silly fat woman' who once again lets herself be fooled by the system and tricked to obey the norms" (Juti 2017) can compromise the budding clout fat activism now has in Finnish society. Focusing on "silly" individuals discredits the aims of fat activism and obfuscates the power it could potentially have as a social movement. Furthermore, when the ambivalence expressed by fat activists is labelled as "silliness" in this way, the activists themselves may choose not to communicate their contradictory thoughts and feelings about fatness. This omission and the ensuing silence can, in turn, become mentally burdensome.

It is important to normalize the experience of ambivalence for two reasons: first, in order to prevent fat activists who experience ambivalence from being silenced as "hypocrites" by others; and second, in order to keep fat activists from self-silencing out of fear of being judged hypocritical. Instead of being trapped in ambivalence, centering it as a normal and expected consequence of living in a culture that hates and fears fatness can shore up ambivalence as a powerful place from which to continue the fight to advance the rights and interests of fat people.

Notes

1. Unfortunately, I was not able to access exact data on column readership; however, the columns have been actively shared on Facebook—barring one, hundreds of times, and on occasion, thousands.
2. The numbers refer to the columns, which I have numbered in chronological order. The original language of the texts is Finnish; I have translated the excerpts.

Acknowledgments

I thank the two anonymous reviewers whose insightful comments helped improve this manuscript.

References

Anonymous. n.d. "Finnish Fatlogic (In Finnish): The Scale Rebellion! [Web Log Comment]." https://www.reddit.com/r/fatlogic/comments/5ncl0n/finnish_fatlogic_in_finnish_the_scale_rebellion/

Ayuso, L. 2001. "I Look FAT in This!" In *Turbo Chicks: Talking Young Feminisms*, edited by A. Mitchell, L. Bryn Rundle, and L. Karaian, 155–61. Toronto: Sumach Press.

Cooper, C. 1998. *Fat and Proud: The Politics of Size*. London: The Women's Press.

Cooper, C. 2008. "*Working Paper WP2008-02. September 2008.*" University of Limerick, Department of Sociology Working Paper Series. Accessed https://ulir.ul.ie/bitstream/handle/10344/3628/Cooper_2008_fat.pdf?sequence=2

Cooper, C. 2009. "Maybe It Should Be Called Fat American Studies?" In *The Fat Studies Reader*, edited by E. Rothblum and S. Solovay, 327–33. New York and London: New York University Press.

Cooper, C. 2010. "Fat Studies: Mapping the Field." *Sociology Compass* 4 (12):1020–34. doi:10.1111/j.1751-9020.2010.00336.x.

Cooper, C. 2016. *Fat Activism: A Radical Social Movement*. Bristol, UK: HammerOn Press.

Cooper, C., and S. Murray. 2012. "Fat Activist Community: A Conversation Piece." *Somatechnics* 2 (1):127–38. doi:10.3366/soma.2012.0045.

Donaghue, N., and A. Clemitshaw. 2012. "'I'm Totally Smart and a Feminist…And yet I Want to Be a Waif': Exploring Ambivalence Towards the Thin Ideal within the Fat Acceptance Movement." *Women's Studies International Forum* 35 (6):415–25. doi:10.1016/j.wsif.2012.07.005.

Gruys, K. 2012. "Does This Make Me Look Fat? Aesthetic Labor and Fat Talk as Emotional Labor in a Women's Plus-Size Clothing Store." *Social Problems* 59 (4):481–500. doi:10.1525/sp.2012.59.4.481.

Hardin, J. 2015. "Christianity, Fat Talk, and Samoan Pastors: Rethinking the Fat-Positive-Fat-Stigma Framework." *Fat Studies* 4 (2):178–96. doi:10.1080/21604851.2015.1015924.

Harjunen, H. 2017. *Neoliberal Bodies and the Gendered Fat Body*. London and New York: Routledge.

Härkönen, J., and P. Räsänen. 2008. "Liikalihavuus, työttömyys ja ansiotaso." *Työelämän tutkimus – Arbetslivsforskning* 6 (1):3–16.

Hsieh, H.-F., and S. E. Shannon. 2005. "Three Approaches to Qualitative Content Analysis." *Qualitative Health Research* 15 (9):1277–88. doi:10.1177/1049732305276687.

Hyttinen, N. 2017, January 11. "Kapina vaakaa vai tervettä järkeä ja kansanterveyttä vastaan, verorahoilla? [Web log post]." Accessed http://nuuttihyttinen.puheenvuoro.uusisuomi.fi/229301-kapina-vaakaa-vai-tervetta-jarkea-ja-kansanterveytta-vastaan-verorahoilla

Jokinen, A., K. Juhila, and E. Suoninen. 1993. *Diskurssianalyysin aakkoset*. Tampere: Vastapaino.

Jutel, A. 2005. "Weighing Health: The Moral Burden of Obesity." *Social Semiotics* 15 (2):113–25. doi:10.1080/10350330500154717.

Juti, M. 2017, June 27. "Läskiaktivisti Vai Vaakakapinallinen? [Web Log Post]." Accessed https://blogit.apu.fi/minna/laskiaktivisti-vai-vaakakapinallinen/

Kauppinen, K., and E. Anttila. 2005. "Onko painolla väliä: Hoikat, lihavat ja normaalipainoiset naiset työelämän murroksessa?" *Työ ja ihminen* 19 (2):239–56.

Kyrölä, K., and H. Harjunen. 2017. "Phantom/Liminal Fat and Feminist Theories of the Body." *Feminist Theory* 18 (2):99–117. doi:10.1177/1464700117700035.

Laapotti, S. 2017. "Ruumiillisuus, lihavuus ja sukupuoli – Mikä ja kuka meitä määrittää? *Tiedonjyvä Jyväskylän yliopiston alumnilehti 2017*." 18–19. Accessed https://issuu.com/universityofjyvaskyla/docs/tiedonjyva_alumninumero_2017_-_smal

LeBesco, K. 2004. *Revolting Bodies? the Struggle to Redefine Fat Identity*. Amherst and Boston, MA: University of Massachusetts Press.

Lehtinen, J. n.d. "Jennyn Elämänmuutos [Landing Page for the Column Series]." Accessed https://yle.fi/aihe/kategoria/vaakakapina/jennyn-elamanmuutos

Lupton, D. 2018. *Fat*. London and New York: Routledge.

Maor, M. 2013a. "'Do I Still Belong Here?' The Body's Boundary Work in the Israeli Fat Acceptance Movement." *Social Movement Studies* 12 (3):280–97. doi:10.1080/14742837.2012.716251.

Maor, M. 2013b. "Becoming the Subject of Your Own Story: Creating Fat-Positive Representations." *Interdisciplinary Humanities* 30 (3):7–22.

McMichael, M. R. 2010. *The Dynamics of Fat Acceptance: Rhetoric and Resistance to the Obesity Epidemic* (Doctoral dissertation, Texas Tech University). Retrieved from https://ttu-ir.tdl.org/ttu-ir/bitstream/handle/2346/ETD-TTU-2010-12-1125/MCMICHAEL-DISSERTATION.pdf?sequence=2

Meleo-Erwin, Z. 2011. "'A Beautiful Show of Strength': Weight Loss and the Fat Activist Self." *Health* 15 (2):188–205. doi:10.1177/1363459310361601.

Meleo-Erwin, Z. 2012. "Disrupting Normal: Toward the 'Ordinary and Familiar' in Fat Politics." *Feminism & Psychology* 22 (3):388–402. doi:10.1177/0959353512445358.

Merimaa, M., and N. Stolt n.d. "Älä mahdu muottiin [Web log post]." Accessed https://ihanaelamys.fi/project/ala-mahdu-muottiin/

Monaghan, L. F., R. Colls, and B. Evans. 2013. "Obesity Discourse and Fat Politics: Research, Critique and Interventions." *Critical Public Health* 23 (3):249–62. doi:10.1080/09581596.2013.814312.

More to Love. n.d. "Plus Mimmi/I Am Peppi [English Description in Right Sidebar]." Accessed http://www.moretolove.fi/

Murray, S. 2005. "(Un/Be)Coming Out? Rethinking Fat Politics." *Social Semiotics* 15 (2):153–63. doi:10.1080/10350330500154667.

Murray, S. 2008. *The 'Fat' Female Body.* New York: Palgrave Macmillan.

Murray, S. 2010. "Doing Politics or Selling Out? Living the Fat Body." *Women's Studies* 34 (3–4):265–77. doi:10.1080/00497870590964165.

Mustajoki, P. 2018, February 26. "Kaloreiden Uhrit Ry. [Web Log Post]." Accessed https://www.perttimustajoki.fi/kaloreiden-uhrit-ry/

Omaheimo, R., (Playwright), and E. Kilkku (Dramaturg). 2016. *Läski. Rasvainen monologi lihavuudesta [Theatrical performance].* Finland: Teatteri Takomo.

Omaheimo, R., and S. Särmä 2017, June 29. "Kuuma läskikeskustelu [Web log post]." Accessed http://hairikot.voima.fi/artikkeli/kuuma-laskikeskustelu/

Orbach, S. 1978. *Fat Is a Feminist Issue: How to Lose Weight Permanently – Without Dieting.* London: Arrow Books.

Owen, L. J. 2015. "Monstrous Freedom: Charting Fat Ambivalence." *Fat Studies* 4 (1):1–13. doi:10.1080/21604851.2014.896186.

Palinkas, L., S. Horwitz, C. Green, J. Wisdom, N. Duan, and K. Hoagwood. 2015. "Purposeful Sampling for Qualitative Data Collection and Analysis in Mixed Method Implementation Research." *Administration and Policy in Mental Health and Mental Health Services Research* 42 (5):533–44. doi:10.1007/s10488-013-0528-y.

Pausé, C. 2015. "Rebel Heart: Performing Fatness Wrong Online." *M/C - A Journal of Media and Culture* 18 (3). Retrieved from http://www.journal.media-culture.org.au/index.php/mcjournal/article/viewArticle/977.

Pausé, C. November 2017. *Fatness, Body Politics, and You: The Role of Fat Ethics in Your Work.* Finland: Visiting lecture at the University of Jyväskylä.

Preckel, K., D. Scheele, M. Eckstein, W. Meier, and R. Hurlemann. 2015. "The Influence of Oxytocin on Volitional and Emotional Ambivalence." *Social Cognitive and Affective Neuroscience* 10 (7):987–93. doi:10.1093/scan/nsu147.

Puhl, R. M., J. D. Latner, K. O'Brien, J. Luedicke, S. Danielsdottir, and M. Forhan. 2015. "A Multinational Examination of Weight Bias: Predictors of Anti-Fat Attitudes across Four Countries." *International Journal of Obesity* 39 (7):1166–73. doi:10.1038/ijo.2015.32.

Read, K. 2017, May 20. "Internalised Fatphobia Is Still Fatphobia [Web Log Post]." Accessed https://fatheffalump.wordpress.com/2017/05/20/internalised-fathphobia-is-still-fatphobia/

Rissanen, A., and P. Mustajoki. 2006. "Lihavuuden ja syömisen psykologiaa." In *Lihavuus: Ongelma ja hoito*, edited by P. Mustajoki, M. Fogelholm, A. Rissanen, and M. Uusitupa, 119–27. Helsinki: Duodecim.

Rose Water Magazine. 2015, March 10. "How the 'Inspiring' Good Fatty Hurts the Body Positive Movement [Web log post]." Accessed https://rosewatermag.com/2015/03/10/how-the-inspiring-good-fatty-hurts-the-body-positive-movement/

Scale Rebellion. n.d. "Vaakakapina. Lopeta laihdutus, aloita elämä [Landing page for the Scale Rebellion]." Accessed https://yle.fi/aihe/vaakakapina

Sieluni silmin. 2018, January 8. "Vastalause kiusaamiselle À la Vaakakapina [Web log post]." Accessed http://www.sielunisilmin.fi/malelifestyle/vaakakapina-venla-palkinto/

"Society". n.d. *WordReference.com Online Language Dictionaries.* Accessed http://www.wordreference.com/definition/society

Solovay, S., and E. Rothblum 2009. *"No Fear of Fat."* Accessed http://chronicle.com/article/No-Fear-of-Fat/49041/

Statistics Finland. 2008. *"1. Vieraita kieliä osaa entistä useampi suomalainen."* Accessed https://www.stat.fi/til/aku/2006/03/aku_2006_03_2008-06-03_kat_001_fi.html

Statistics Finland. 2017. *"Matkapuhelin yhä suositumpi laite internetin käyttöön – Käyttötarkoitukset monipuolistuvat."* Accessed https://www.stat.fi/til/sutivi/2017/13/sutivi_2017_13_2017-11-22_tie_001_fi.html

Tahvanainen, H. 2017, January 11. "Vaakakapinat ovat monelle vaarallista peliä [Web log post]." Accessed https://www.karjalainen.fi/mielipiteet/mielipiteet/kolumnit/item/127401-vaakakapinat-ovat-monelle-vaarallista-pelia

Vatsamielenosoitus. n.d. "Vatsamielenosoitus kauneusihanteille [Blog landing page]." Accessed https://vatsamielenosoitus.wordpress.com/

Wann, M. 1998. *Fat!So?: Because You Don't Have to Apologize for Your Size!* Berkeley, CA: Ten Speed Press.

White, F. R. 2014. "Fat/Trans: Queering the Activist Body." *Fat Studies* 3 (2):86–100. doi:10.1080/21604851.2014.889489.

Yle. 2017. *"Laihuuden ihannoinnin järkyttävä tulos: 84 prosenttia naisista tyytymättömiä painoonsa."* Accessed https://yle.fi/uutiset/3-9385699

Yle. 2018. *"Vaakakapina - kansanliike, joka mursi pikadieettien vallan."* Accessed https://yle.fi/aihe/artikkeli/2018/01/16/vaakakapina-kansanliike-joka-mursi-pikadieettien-vallan

Yle. n.d. *"This Is Yle."* Accessed https://yle.fi/aihe/artikkeli/about-yle/this-is-yle

Ylönen, E. 2017, October 1. "A-Teema ja lihava Suomi [Web log post]." Accessed http://queenofeverything.fitfashion.fi/2017/10/01/teema-ja-lihava-suomi/

Zembylas, M. 2012. "The Politics of Fear and Empathy: Emotional Ambivalence in 'Host' Children and Youth Discourses about Migrants in Cyprus." *Ethnic and Racial Studies* 33 (8):1372–91. doi:10.1080/14675986.2012.701426.

"You will face discrimination": Fatness, motherhood, and the medical profession

Jennifer Lee

ABSTRACT

This is an autoethnographic article that explores the intersection of fatness, pregnancy, motherhood, health and diabetes, and interaction with the medical profession. The autoethnographic approach used includes both written stories and photographic narrative. There have been times when my fat body has been seen by the medical profession as barren, incapable, and excessive and also times when I didn't know whether I could trust a medical opinion to be objective, because I inhabit a fat body. I discuss medical and cultural assumptions about a fat woman's ability to conceive, oppressive medical policies, such as how much weight a fat woman "should" gain in pregnancy and what she "should" eat according to medical guidelines. In addition, I document the complicating factor of having diabetes and the hypermonitoring of blood sugar and "dieting" to keep a baby safe, and the return of guilt about eating "the wrong things." I tell these stories to illuminate what the medicalization of fatness, pregnancy, and early motherhood have been like, including the effect it had on my ability to practice fat acceptance. The article is framed by both scholarly and fat activist approaches to the discussion of fat embodiment, pregnancy, childbirth, and breastfeeding, in an attempt to expose discrimination and oppression of fat women's bodies within the medical field. I consider the question: How can a fat woman have a voice during pregnancy and into motherhood?

Introduction

This is an autoethnographic article about my experience of conception, pregnancy, childbirth, and breastfeeding as a fat woman. The methods used to explore my changing experiences of fatness and motherhood in this article are journal writing, photography (see Figure 1), and critical essay writing, which were conducted across four years. These private narratives are framed with reference to how fatness is treated in western culture. Within my creative writing discipline area, I have also researched writing about taboo and trauma, and the initial shame associated with telling such private stories. I have long believed in the value of peeling back the layers of shame, to

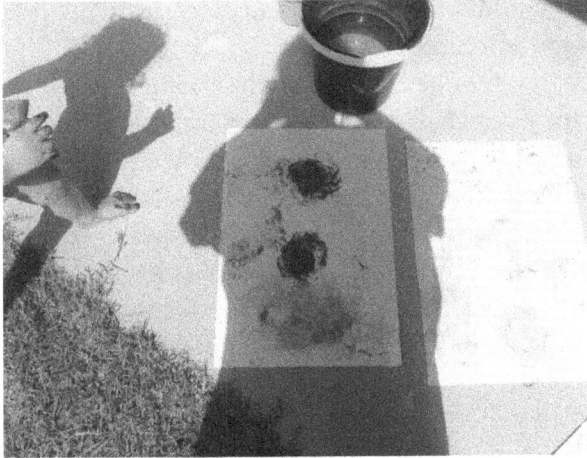

Figure 1. Mother and daughter.

reveal, and question what is hidden beneath. In this process, a strong voice can grow, and autoethnography can give this voice an audience.

I consider autoethnography a methodology but also a way of positioning readership, enhancing the relationship between writer and reader, and defining reader expectation. There is therapeutic value (for readers), and also vulnerability, for the writer, in revealing stories to the world. Autoethnography positions the writer and reveals the distance from the events or experiences or identity being discussed in the piece. Autoethnography can also influence and infiltrate the life of the writer – to live more reflectively, and to consciously consider experiences and how they could be more than a source of pain or discomfort. Stigmatization, prejudice, rejection, and self-hatred separate a person from engaging in the world in meaningful ways, cause social isolation, and are related to depression. Autoethnography, sharing stories and vulnerability, is essentially connecting to the world, and is a hopeful act. This is particularly important for a stigmatized group.

There are other autoethnographic accounts relating to fatness that have emerged in recent years. These accounts range from discussing fat and weight loss and conflicting social messages (Leith 2016) to feminist narratives that refuse the perspective of women who are dieting or unhappy being fat (Smailes 2014) to coming out as fat (Pausé 2012). I have at times focused on autoethnography around fat and queer identities, and sexuality (Lee 2014, 2015a). Other fat autoethnography links the personal experiences and intersectionality of the authors with the societal and cultural phenomena of "obesity" and weight loss (Johnson and Eaves 2013). A recent powerful autoethnography is Pausé's work on being denied residency in New Zealand based on her body mass index (Pausé 2018), which she also discussed in a collaborative autoethnography we wrote together (Lee and Pausé 2016). These autoethnographic accounts include describing cultural experiences, and the personal within cultural experiences, signaling that it is autoethnography, not simply autobiography.

It is important to consider the hierarchical nature of some research, even some ethnographic research, if it is methodologically designed and performed by a researcher of a less "othered" or stigmatized identity. It is useful to consider ethical considerations around methodology, the assumptions being made, which questions are asked, and the discussion of data (for example, the "obesity paradox" can only exist if it is assumed that "obesity" is bad for you).

The importance and significance of autoethnography in fat studies includes reclaiming a voice in a publication field where fat voices are most often excluded from "obesity" research, and excluded from the development of methodology on reporting "successful weight loss narratives." Our voices need to be present in the research, not just as quoted people who are interviewed, but also as the researchers who frame our own stories, our experiences, and how they relate to the existing research. Autoethnography can shift the hierarchy and put the research and the story/voice back into the hands of the affected group.

In addition, writing stories for stigmatized groups who experience violence and hate is important. In the case of fat people, this violence and hate takes many forms, including being entrenched in the medical profession. Tony Adams, in the *Handbook of Autoethnography* (2015), discusses ostracism, pain, and suicide around stigmatized queer identities. He found the intimate, personal, and relational work in autoethnography to be important for queer people who were being harmed by ignorance and hate.

I am an Anglo-Australian cisgendered queer academic in my early 40s. I grew up in the lower socioeconomic multicultural western suburbs of Melbourne. I had to learn to fit in when a wealthy friend of the family saw my potential and paid for me to attend a private secondary school. My education includes undergraduate study with honors, a teaching qualification, and a PhD. I am aware of the privilege I was born with and the privilege I gathered through financial support and education. This privilege is partly why I have been invited to speak to the media about fat issues, and I have selectively done so. In the stories in this autoethnography, I was in a heterosexual relationship, and, as a cisgendered woman, I didn't have to navigate or reveal my queerness to medical professionals.

In this article, I discuss medical and cultural assumptions about conception, pregnancy, birth, and mothering, and I document the complicating factor of having type 2 diabetes. I have written and published autoethnography that focuses on the interaction between my diabetes and fatness in the past (Lee 2012, 2015b). This article is framed by both scholarly and fat activist approaches to the discussion of fat embodiment, pregnancy, childbirth and breastfeeding, and the experiences of fat mothers. The sections demonstrate the stereotyping, discrimination and assumptions made about fat women. At times, the hysteria about "obesity" overrode my voice and wishes. I acknowledge my privilege, desire to control the outcomes, high expectations of myself, prenatal and postnatal anxiety depression, and the sense that I lost my voice. Finally, I discuss fat acceptance, celebration and defiance, and the body-positive approach I take with my daughter. Throughout the article, I consider the question: How can a fat woman have a voice during pregnancy and into motherhood?

Stereotyping, discrimination, and hysteria: Pre-pregnancy

I had heard how fat women, especially "morbidly obese" women like me, would have trouble conceiving a baby. I had been diagnosed with type 2 diabetes when I was 34 years old, and I had difficulty coming to terms with that, especially because there tends to be hysteria around diabetes as an illness. I think of it as a "death-fatty-diabesity-scary-horror-music" illness, in that it is presented as one of the worst illness one can have. This meant that I delayed trying to conceive for a further two to three years.

At times, I keep an audio journal, meaning if I don't have time to write it down and there's something I want to express or keep on record, I record it on my phone. Here is a transcription recording from 2013, before I conceived:

> After Aquaporko [fat synchronized swim team] practice we had nice coffee and food and chatted. We talked about pregnancy and I was advised to 'go private, go private' in order to choose my own medical specialists, but I feel like I have a right to go through the public system and to be respected or demand respect or demand not to see that particular person or have that person treat me if they're rude to me.

When I decided to get advice about conceiving, I was referred to the diabetes pregnancy clinic at the Royal Women's Hospital in Melbourne. They started me on metformin and insulin and studied my results to ensure my blood sugars were within normal range before conception, as they stated that out of control blood sugar numbers can lead to miscarriage, large babies, and congenital issues. I began measuring, obsessing, and achieving what the endocrinologist called "A+ grades" all the way through pregnancy with blood sugars. However, the self-monitoring reminded me of dieting and I judged myself through the process. The levels of my anxiety were high and untreated.

It was around this time of preconception that I was introduced to the diabetes clinic dietician who was very fatphobic and I never returned to see her. She interrogated me about what I ate, and didn't listen to me when I spoke about not wanting to measure my food and potentially trigger problematic eating behaviors. Anti-fat attitudes are well documented in medical professionals, students, and nurses (Berryman et al. 2006; Persky and Eccleston 2011; Poon and Tarrant 2009; Sabin, Marini, and Nosek 2012; Schwartz et al. 2003; Setchell et al. 2014; Stone and Werner 2012). I wrote a long complaint letter that was addressed by the hospital (to read more about this, refer to Lee and Pause 2016). I had been warned by a Health At Every Size (HAES) dietician in the year before, "you will face discrimination." George Parker mirrors this when she states:

> ...women classified as 'obese' [are framed as] either willingly risking their baby's health, or lacking the knowledge or self-discipline to make the required 'lifestyle changes' to reduce the risks their bodies pose to the developing fetus. In keeping with this individual framing, the solution lies in following 'expert advice' and making the recommended changes to diet and physical activity (2014).

However, in ignoring my voice, and focusing only on weight loss, I was not able to trust this dietician's advice on any aspect of my pregnancy. It would be worthwhile for medical professionals to remember that, to treat or enact change in a patient's life, or indeed to monitor a pregnancy, the patient has to feel able to return to the treatment office. If the patient is too traumatized to do so, then a medical professional's opportunity to treat the patient is lost.

Assumptions, risk, and anxiety: Pregnancy

For much of my pregnancy, I read and researched fatness, childbirth options, and medical assumptions. My psychologist suggested I stop doing this because it fed into my anxiety. However, I felt that I couldn't trust my care to medical professionals, considering their assumptions and prejudices about the risk of my fatness to my pregnancy (McPhail et al. 2016). I wanted to know enough to be able to have a say in my treatment, and in what was best for my unborn child.

Although I was in the public medical system, I flatly refused to return to the first obstetrician after she immediately said, "You'll be having a C-section." I had read accounts of the bias toward recommending C-sections to fat women and the evidence that "obese" women should be given access to individual decision making based on their health risks, not based on a routine policy (Abenhaim and Benjamin 2011; Homer et al. 2011; Subramaniam et al. 2014; Wispelwey and Sheiner 2012). These studies show that a higher number of "obese" mothers have C-sections because they are told they have to have one or they will put their baby at risk (McPhail et al. 2016).

I also refused to return to the second obstetrician after he recommended dieting to keep to a certain level of weight gain. In 2009, the Institute of Medicine in the United States released new pregnancy weight gain guidelines (Einerson et al. 2011). I gained 13 kg during pregnancy, which fits into what those with a "normal body mass index" are supposed to gain, but according to guidelines, which the second obstetrician quoted at me, I should only have gained between 5 and 9 kg (11–20 pounds).

I asked to see a third obstetrician that a midwife had recommended to me as "pro-natural birth, she used to run a natural birthing center, and has a good bedside manner" in the diabetes pregnancy clinic. This obstetrician was indeed wonderful, and encouraged my questions throughout pregnancy. She suggested I could weigh myself each fortnight in the hospital before my appointment and let her know if there was a big jump in weight, so she could check for any medical issues related to that. Her trust in me, and the fact that she listened to my concerns, was probably the single biggest positive aspect to her treatment for me.

Despite my weight gain, no one knew I was pregnant until about the eighth month, unless I told them. As a fat woman, I didn't develop that traditionally seen pregnant stomach silhouette. I still had a "double" stomach, it never became one big round shape (see Figure 2). Some of the joy, in my case, of waiting for a new person, was dampened by this expectation I had of looking identifiably pregnant in the traditional sense. But I viewed pictures of other fat pregnant women at "the well-rounded mama" (Vireday 2013) blog and it helped to see a range of other fat pregnant bodies. Furber and McGowan (2011), scholars in midwifery and women's health in the United Kingdom, discuss this experience as quite common for "obese" and pregnant women. This is partly because only the traditional pregnant shape is seen in the media.

I developed prenatal depression and anxiety, especially during the hormone-drenched first three months when I was physically sick as well. This went

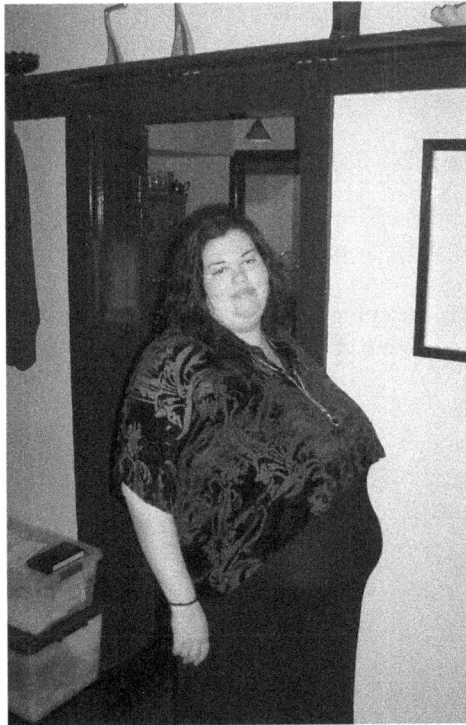

Figure 2. My pregnancy shape.

untreated at first, because, as previously stated, the first obstetrician looked at me when I was seven weeks pregnant, and without examining me, discussing my medical history, or asking about my birth preferences, announced, "You'll be having a C-section." When I asked her if this was because of being fat, she said "You're obsessed with the fat issue, not me. I've been on every diet in the book, I can't talk." I never got an answer about why she pronounced that because I refused, in tears, to return to her. My anxiety and fear of discrimination increased. I felt, at this stage, that I didn't have a voice.

High expectations and postnatal depression: The birth

I had been treated with respect by the third obstetrician, and by the endocrinologist, although she made classist remarks several times, which reminded me, I am a fat white cis-gendered middle-class educated woman, albeit with working-class family roots. I have no doubt that I received better care from her at times because I was educated, and I have a PhD. She therefore believed what I said and could relate to me.

The following is an extract from an audio journal, day 10 after my daughter's birth, on January 27, 2014.

> Been home a couple of days now after a week in hospital with an infection.
>
> I resisted the medicalization for so long but in the end, I realized that I needed it. And when you're induced, the contractions are full on, it's an early induction, it's highly likely to end in a C-section, and I felt that if I avoided certain measures, I could avoid that.

Audio journal, January 27, 2014:

> Then they say the baby's heart rate is dropping, you might have to have a c-section, and I felt like, I've done acupuncture, I've been to the osteopath, I've done exercises for avoiding posterior position, I drank raspberry leaf tea, I did meditation, internal massage, breathing exercises, practice labor positions, hip jiggling, all of that, and in the end, none of it could trump the fact that she wasn't in a good

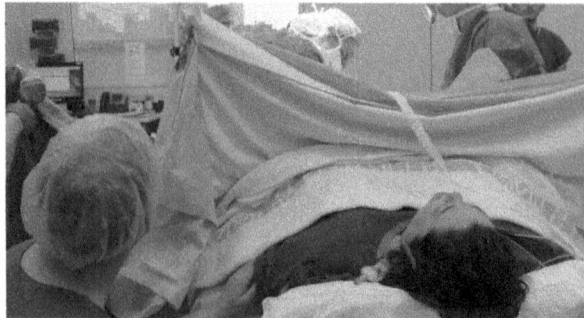

Figure 3. Having a Caesarean Section after 36 hr of induced labor.

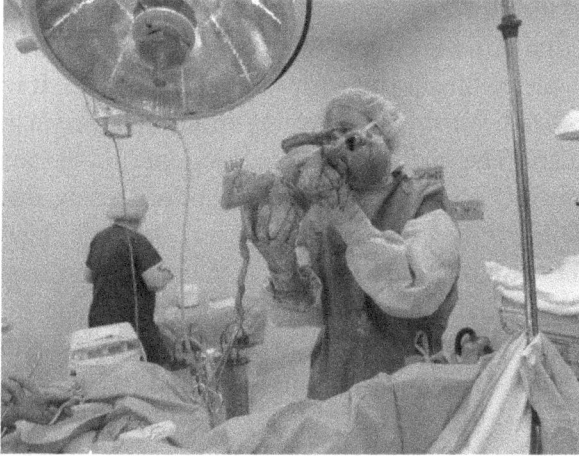

Figure 4. My daughter's birth.

position, and labor didn't progress beyond 4 cm. Birthing, like health, like fatness, is not something I could control.

My daughter's heart rate dropped again so there was an emergency C-section (see Figures 3, 4 and 5).

I thought that if I controlled that process and stayed away from the medicalized model that treats fat women with disdain, I could feel empowered and happy and have that vaginal birth. Instead, the no-drugs guide I'd planned before the labor left me feeling traumatized, disempowered, and without a voice. Despite repeatedly asking for drugs during the relentless contractions, the midwives and doula ignored my requests and stuck to my prebirth plan. After the birthing process, I realized that actually what I needed was just a voice in deciding on my treatment during the birth process.

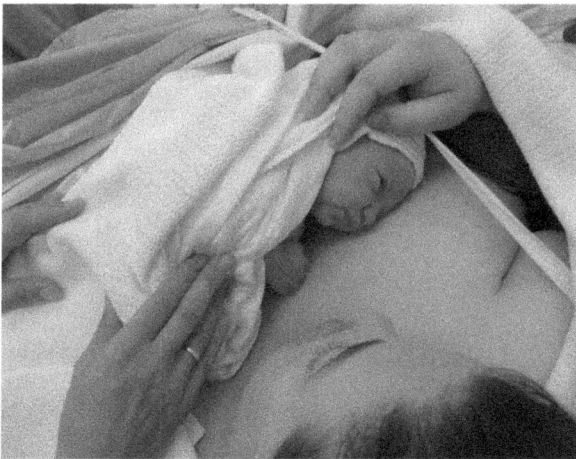

Figure 5. My daughter and I just after the birth.

I had so many medical interventions that I went four days without any sleep at all. After this period of no sleep and major surgery recovery, they discovered an infection, which started three to four days after the C-section. It was at that point that my daughter's father insisted on sleeping on a trundle bed in my room to help me during the night. The midwife got permission for him to stay the night once I dropped my daughter under the covers during breastfeeding, due to exhaustion. My daughter's father wanted to assist in any way he could, however fathers or partners were not encouraged to be present in the hospital overnight in those first days after childbirth (see Figure 6 where he baths our daughter).

Reflecting on this now, I realize the breastfeeding schedule the hospital had me on contributed to the unrealistic and high expectations I had of myself.

These expectations were directly related to what I wanted my fat body to be able to do. I thought, "Just because I'm fat, doesn't mean I'm unfit." My body can achieve a natural childbirth. But an induction is not a natural process. In fact, my fatness led to a sense of wanting to prove myself able in labor, of setting too-high expectations, of then seeing myself as a failure, which in turn contributed to postnatal depression.

My daughter became very ill with a life-threatening infection at 28 days old. I was medicated for depression for the first time. In addition, I read a French study that found when grandmothers had postnatal depression, their daughters are much more likely to suffer from postnatal depression (Séjourné et al. 2011, 121). My mother suffered from untreated postnatal depression. She was also a slim woman until after I was born, when her dieting and my father's fat shaming of her began, and I have wondered about the effect of her body hatred beginning with her pregnancy and weight gain around that time.

I received some relief when a Lactation Consultant and a General Medical Practitioner friend who practices Health At Every Size® advised me to spend

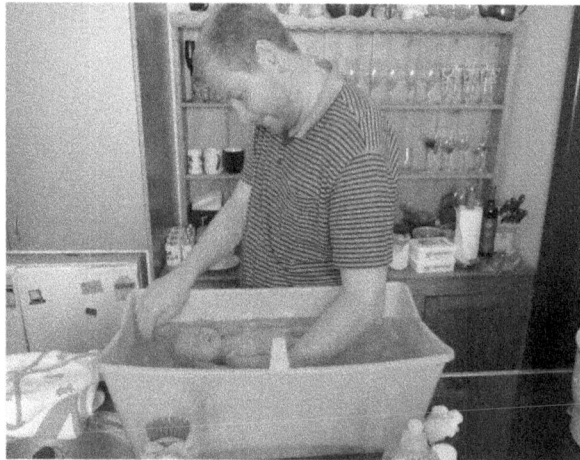

Figure 6. My daughter's father bathing her.

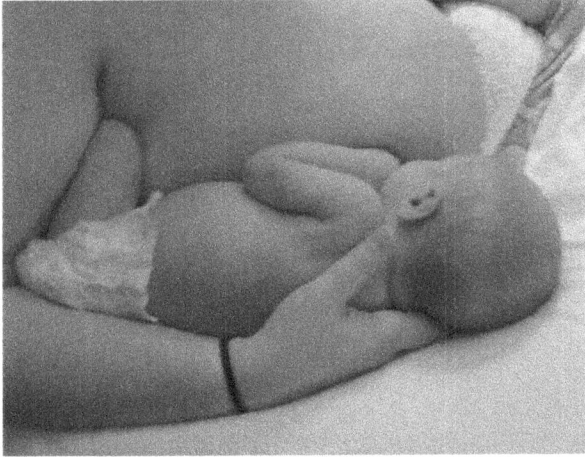

Figure 7. In Australia, this is referred to as "football" style breastfeeding—I couldn't breastfeed the "usual" way due to my size.

less time pumping milk, and to supplement with a bottle of formula. My friend could probably see that my 16 hours of sitting in the chair, trying to make enough food for my daughter, was not helping my mental health.

Diets for baby: breastfeeding

A maternal health nurse, upon seeing my baby's growth rate, prescribed a diet for her at seven months of age (see Figure 10). My daughter would have screamed in hunger. I was told to remove the one bottle of supplemented formula I was giving her per day, and just breastfeed her(see Figures 7, 8 and 9).

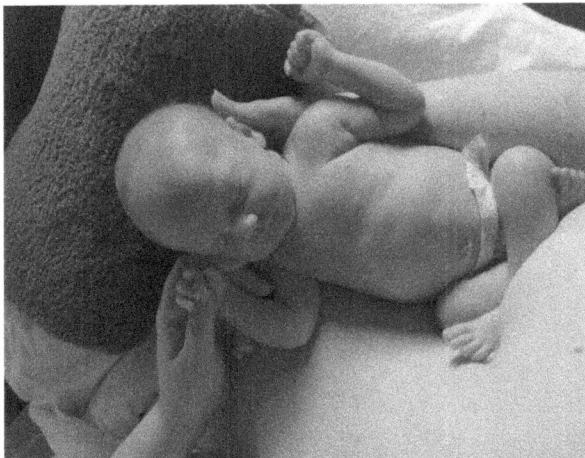

Figure 8. Resting after breastfeeding.

The following is from an audio journal recording on February 24, 2014.

She's cluster feeding in chunks again. They talk about growth spurts and cluster feeding and she has been doing it since day one and it's now five and a half weeks. I'm spending 14–16 hours in an armchair either breastfeeding or pumping every last drop for her to drink.

Audio recording, February 24, 2014:

I can't seem to breastfeed lying down. I am buggered at this point. I know her body was starving when my placenta failed, and now she is catching up – just like a dieter who then needs to eat, and whose body wants to get back to where they were previously [as I had read in Bacon's HAES, 2008].

May Friedman (2015) rightly argues that "The policing of fat children and their parents rest on two commonsense medical truths that are central to the rhetoric of 'obesity': first, fat is unhealthy, and, second, fat is reversible. These arguments are at the center of cases that view fat children as evidence of medical neglect" (18).

I would also argue that fat mothers are seen as having children with the potential to be fat. In my case, they assumed that the fat mother was over-feeding her child. My daughter was growing exponentially; therefore, they assumed she was on track to keep growing exponentially and to become fat. In fact, in fat studies we know that putting her on a diet would most likely have eventually led to potential eating disorders, potential bingeing and future weight gain, with further fatness (Bacon 2008).

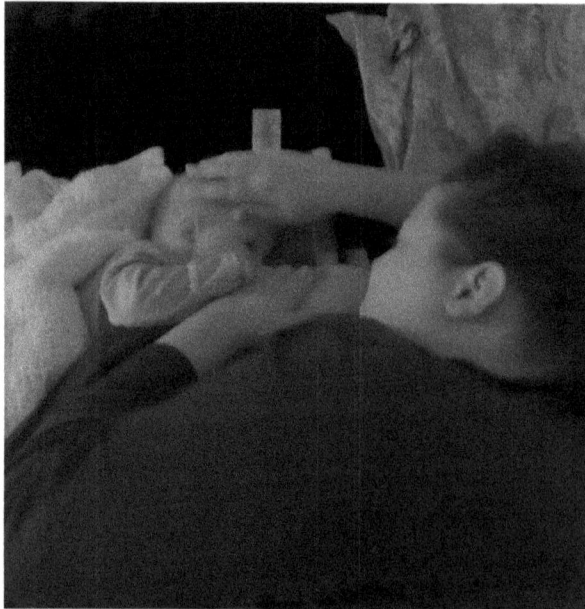

Figure 9. Finally, at 5 months, I learned how to breastfeed lying down. The problem was the instructions given to me at the hospital didn't work for a fat body. In the end, I read some fat blogs and experimented.

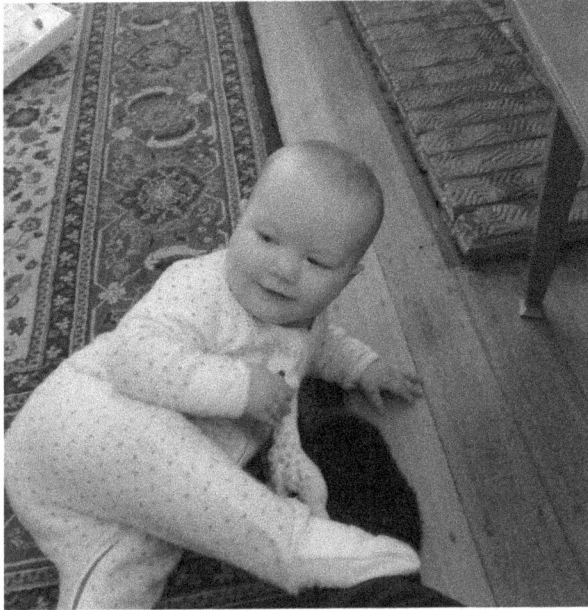

Figure 10. A maternal health nurse advised me to restrict my daughter's eating around this time.

Fat acceptance, celebration, and defiance: Mothering a toddler

I was having a shower with my daughter and I soaped her up and then rinsed it off. She then wanted to wash my stomach, so she soaped up her hands and rubbed them all over my stomach happily. After being dried, she was dancing naked—kicking one leg up, her "dog wag" dance, where she copies our miniature dachshund, and her twirling dance.

I threw off the towel and did some of her dance moves as we sang, and added some moves from the couple of years when I did belly dance lessons. I pushed my stomach in and out and moved the fat in a snake-like way. She was fascinated and tried (unsuccessfully) to do it. I then deliberately jiggled my fat—legs, belly, breasts, and she watched for a bit, then danced again. Then, I wrapped myself up in the towel again and went to get dressed. I turned the heater up so she could spend more time naked.

I grew up seeing my mother and her mother naked, and they would proclaim how ugly they were, how much they hated parts of their bodies—parts, as if we are cuts of meat to be sliced up and picked over—never whole women to be loved. Then, they would pack themselves up into girdles, to hide their stomachs in particular.

Since she was a baby, I have massaged my daughter with baby oil, with her naked and me partly naked, in the summer (see Figure 11).

As she has grown older, she requests a "fassage" before bed. I give her foot and leg massages and we talk about everything legs can do. They can walk, run, jump, dance, kick (yes, but we don't kick people or the dog), climb, and swim. This

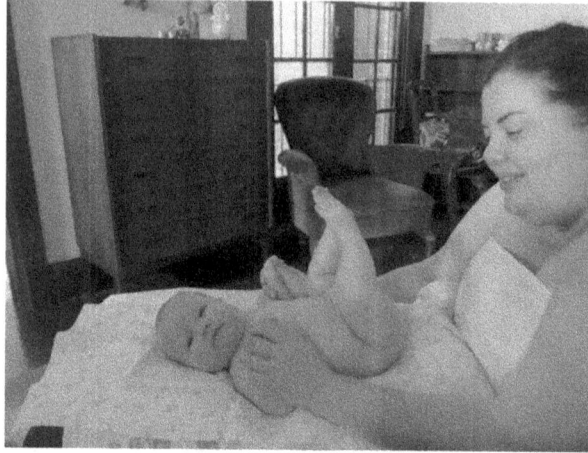

Figure 11. Me massaging my daughter.

comes out of my reading on girls who focus on what their bodies are capable of achieving rather than solely on their appearance being less likely to suffer from negative body image or fat hatred (Halliwell 2015 & Andrew, Tiggemann, and Clark 2016).

I think about the tight control on my food intake as a child, my binge eating from when I was four years old, my first diet when I was eight years old, and in contrast, the more relaxed approach to my daughter's food and eating, the natural balance she finds, the lack of mystery and obsession around "junk" or "chocolate."

I feel "fat defiant" when I think about raising a daughter who can see her mother jiggle her fat in a naked dance, wear a swimsuit to the beach, eat chocolate without saying "I shouldn't be eating this," and talk about all the great things our bodies are capable of. "Fat defiance" is raising my daughter differently (see Figure 12).

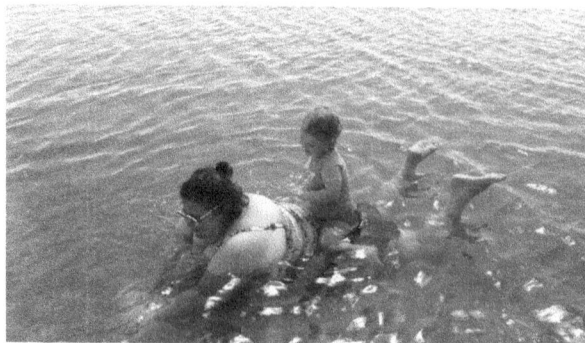

Figure 12. Wearing swimsuits at the beach with my daughter. My mother never swam with us as children because she hated her fat body too much to wear a swimsuit.

Conclusion

I think about my experience as a fat activist and fat studies scholar, someone who actively practices fat positivity, "fat yoga" (Harry 2018), and HAES. I think about how difficult my experience of pre-pregnancy, pregnancy, and motherhood has been with my fat body, even though I had access to information, a network of fat activist friends, and a fat acceptance history. I still experienced shame, negativity, silencing, and pre- and postnatal depression and anxiety. It is a challenge to imagine how difficult it would be for a fat woman who believes the narratives about her body and self-blame.

This notion that a pregnant woman is risking her child's life just by existing as a fat woman (McPhail et al. 2016) is prejudiced, and, I would even say, a form of emotional torture. I would like to see fat women treated with respect and given a voice in their treatment, not simply expected to conform to a particular weight, but for there to be a focus on their mental wellbeing as well as physical health and impact on the fetus. Their mental health and happiness should be considered in the equation, rather than the majority of the focus being on the fetus, which leads to the mother feeling like a vessel who is putting her potential child at risk.

In addition, medical professionals could be more aware of the high expectations that pregnant women and mothers place on themselves, often drawn from society's high expectations of mothers. Instead of reinforcing these expectations, they could encourage pregnant women to seek help, to express their fears, and to reassure them that they will receive compassion. This isn't just about fat motherhood, but when fat women are told their bodies are to blame for any negative outcome in pregnancy, and they are shamed, that shame leads to hiding and silence, and in my case contributed to anxiety and depression.

I was invited to speak about my experiences with student doctors at the University of Melbourne Medical School conference in 2017. I presented some of the material in this article, and I was later emailed by several students, thanking me for changing their views on fat patients, and telling me that they hadn't been exposed to these ideas in the rest of their medical training. I believe that fat studies scholars can impact the treatment of future pregnant women and mothers by continuing to tell our stories, and by encouraging more diverse fat voices.

Disclosure statement

No potential conflict of interest was reported by the author.

References

Abenhaim, HA, and A Benjamin. 2011. "Higher Caesarean Section Rates in Women with Higher Body Mass Index: Are We Managing Labour Differently?" *Journal of Obstetrics and Gynaecology Canada* 33 (5):443–48. doi:10.1016/S1701-2163(16)34876-9

Adams, TE. 2015. "Introduction: Coming to Know Autoethnography as More than a Method." In *Handbook of Autoethnography*, edited by S Holman Jones, TE Adams, and C Ellis, 17–47. New York: Taylor and Francis.

Andrew, R, M Tiggemann, and L Clark. 2016. "Predictors and Health-Related Outcomes of Positive Body Image in Adolescent Girls: A Prospective Study." *Developmental Psychology* 52 (3):463–74. doi:10.1037/dev0000095

Bacon, L. 2008. *Health at Every Size: The Surprising Truth about Your Weight*. Texas, USA: Benbella books.

Berryman, DE, GM Dubale, DS Manchester, and R Mittelstaedt. 2006. "Dietetics Students Possess Negative Attitudes toward Obesity Similar to Nondietetics Students." *Journal of the American Dietetic Association* 106:1678–82. doi: 10.1016/j.jada.2006.07.012.

Einerson, BD, JK Huffman, NB Istwan, DJ Rhea, and SD Joy. 2011. "New Gestational Weight Gain Guidelines: An Observational Study of Pregnancy Outcomes in Obese Women." *Obesity* 19:12. doi: 10.1038/oby.2010.204.

Friedman, M. 2015. "Mother Blame, Fat Shame and Moral Panic: "Obesity" and Child Welfare." *Fat Studies: an Interdisciplinary Journal of Body Weight and Society* 4 (1):14–27. doi:10.1080/21604851.2014.927209

Furber, C, and L McGowan. 2011. "A Qualitative Study of the Experiences of Women Who are Obese and Pregnant in the UK." *Midwifery* 27:4. doi: 10.1016/j.midw.2011.02.004.

Halliwell, E. 2015. "Future Directions for Positive Body Image Research." *Body Image* 14:177–89. doi: 10.1016/j.bodyim.2015.03.003.

Harry, S 2018. "Fat Yoga." Accessed December 7, 2018. https://www.fatyoga.com.au/.

Homer, CS, JJ Kurinczuk, P Spark, P Brocklehurst, and M Knight. 2011. "Planned Vaginal Delivery or Planned Caesarean Delivery in Women with Extreme Obesity." *BJOG* 118 (4):480–87. doi:10.1111/j.1471-0528.2010.02832.x

Johnson, C.R.S, and C.L Eaves. 2013. "An Ounce of Time, a Pound of Responsibilities and a Ton of Weight to Lose: An Autoethnographic Journey of Barriers, Message Adherence and the Weight-Loss Process." *Public Relations Inquiry* 2 (1):95–116. doi:10.1177/2046147X12460949

Lee, J. 2012. "Not Just a Type: Diabetes, Fat and Fear." *Somatechnics* 2 (1):80–83. doi:10.3366/soma.2012.0041

Lee, J. 2014. "Flaunting Fat: Sex with the Lights On." In *Queering Fat Embodiment*, edited by C Pausé, J Wykes, and S Murray, 89–96. Surrey, England: Ashgate.

Lee, J. 2015a. "Hidden and Forbidden: Alter Egos, Invisibility Cloaks and Psychic Fat Suits." In *Fat Sex: New Directions in Theory and Activism*, edited by H Hester and C Walters, 101–14. Surrey, England: Ashgate.

Lee, J. 2015b. "All the Way from (B)Lame to (A)Cceptance: Diabetes, Health and Fat Activism." In *The Politics of Size*, edited by R Chastain, vol. 2, 63–74. California, USA: Praeger.

Lee, J, and C Pausé 2016. "Stigma in Practice: Barriers to Health for Fat Women." *Frontiers in Psychology* 7. doi:10.3389/fpsyg.2016.02063/full>.

Leith, V. 2016. "An Autoethnography of Fat and Weight Loss: Becoming the BwO with Deleuze and Guattari." *Sociological Research Online* 21:3. doi: 10.5153/sro.3971.

McPhail, D, A Bombak, P Ward, and J Allison. 2016. "'Wombs at Risk, Wombs as Risk: Fat Women's Experiences of Reproductive Care." *Fat Studies: an Interdisciplinary Journal of Body Weight and Society* 5 (2):98–115. doi:10.1080/21604851.2016.1143754

Parker, G. 2014. "Mothers at Large: Responsibilizing the Pregnant Self for the "Obesity Epidemic"." *Fat Studies: an Interdisciplinary Journal of Body Weight and Society* 3:2. doi: 10.1080/21604851.2014.889491.

Pausé, C. 2012. "Live to Tell: Coming Out as Fat." *Somatechnics* 2 (1):42–56. doi:10.3366/soma.2012.0038

Pausé, C. 2018. "Frozen: A Fat Tale of Immigration." *Fat Studies: an Interdisciplinary Journal of Body Weight and Society* 8:1.

Persky, S, and CP Eccleston. 2011. "Medical Student Bias and Care Recommendations for an Obese versus Non-Obese Virtual Patient." *International Journal of Obesity* 35:728–35. doi: 10.1038/ijo.2010.173.

Poon, MY, and M Tarrant. 2009. "Obesity: Attitudes of Undergraduate Student Nurses and Registered Nurses." *Journal of Clinical Nursing* 18:2355–65. doi: 10.1111/j.1365-2702.2008.02709.x.

Sabin, JA, M Marini, and BA Nosek. 2012. "Implicit and Explicit Anti-Fat Bias among a Large Sample of Medical Doctors by BMI, Race/Ethnicity and Gender." *PMC* 7:11.

Schwartz, MB, HO Chambliss, KD Brownell, SN Blair, and C Billington. 2003. "Weight Bias among Health Professionals Specializing in Obesity." *Obesity Research* 11:1033–39. doi: 10.1038/oby.2003.142.

Séjourné, N, J Alba, M Onorrus, N Goutaudier, and H Chabrol. 2011. "Intergenerational Transmission of Postpartum Depression." *Journal of Reproductive and Infant Psychology* 29 (2):115–24. doi:10.1080/02646838.2010.551656

Setchell, J, B Watson, L Jones, M Gard, and K Briffa. 2014. "Physiotherapists Demonstrate Weight Stigma: A Cross-Sectional Survey of Australian Physiotherapists." *Journal of Physiotherapy* 60:157–62. doi: 10.1016/j.jphys.2014.06.020.

Smailes, S. 2014. "Negotiating and Navigating My Fat Body – Feminist Autoethnographic Encounters." *Athenea Digital* 14:4.

Stone, O, and P Werner. 2012. "Israeli Dietitians' Professional Stigma Attached to Obese Patients." *Qualitative Health Research* 22:768–76. doi: 10.1177/1049732311431942.

Subramaniam, A, VC Jauk, AR Goss, MD Alvarez, CS Reese, and RK Edwards. 2014. "Mode of Delivery in Women with Class III Obesity: Planned Cesarean Compared to Induction of Labor." *American Journal of Obstetrics and Gynecology* 211 (6):700. doi:10.1016/j.ajog.2014.06.045

Vireday, P. 2013. "The Well-Rounded Mama Blog." Accessed June 24, 2016. wellrounded mama.blogspot.com.

Wispelwey, BP, and E Sheiner. 2012. "Cesarean Delivery in Obese Women: A Comprehensive Review." *Journal of Maternal-Fetal and Neonatal Medicine* 26 (6):547–51. doi:10.3109/14767058.2012.745506

Rock and Rolls: Exploring Body Positivity at Girls Rock Camp

Trisha L. Crawshaw

ABSTRACT

Size scholars routinely discuss the negative effects of fat stigma within youth culture. For example, fat kids are more likely to be bullied than their thinner peers, increasing their risk for depression, loneliness, anxiety, and behavior problems. These studies, however, do not adequately address kids' active resistance to fatphobia and size discrimination. In this chapter, I highlight the importance of kids' resistance work at Girls Rock Camp. Pulling from my own experiences as a (fat) camp counselor, I explore the different ways campers push-back against fat stereotypes. While this push-back creates dialogue around size privilege and oppression, organizational obstacles for fat bodies result in conflicting messages about body positivity. Kids challenge size discrimination on an interpersonal level by showing their stomachs, writing anti-shame lyrics, and criticizing unrealistic beauty standards. Adult volunteers, though, continue to navigate organizational sizeism through inaccessible seating, a culture of fat talk, and anti-fat emotional labor. I argue that while Girls Rock Camp indeed helps kids fight against fat prejudice within youth culture, it simultaneously privileges thin adult bodies at an organizational level.

There are fifteen young campers sitting in a large semi-circle. Some are in chairs, but most are splayed out on the hard, tiled floor. It is the second day of Girls Rock Camp – a music education program for girls and gender-nonconforming kids – and I am leading a workshop on media literacy (Figure 1).

"What does the media tell us about our bodies?" I ask the room full of kids, ages eight to sixteen-years-old.

I call on the first hand that shoots into the air.

"Like, you have to have a really skinny waist and then your hips and stuff have to go like this," the camper answers, as her hands pantomime an hourglass figure.

"Yeah," another camper adds. "Otherwise, you can't wear crop tops!"

"WHOA," I interrupt, "Anyone can wear a crop top."

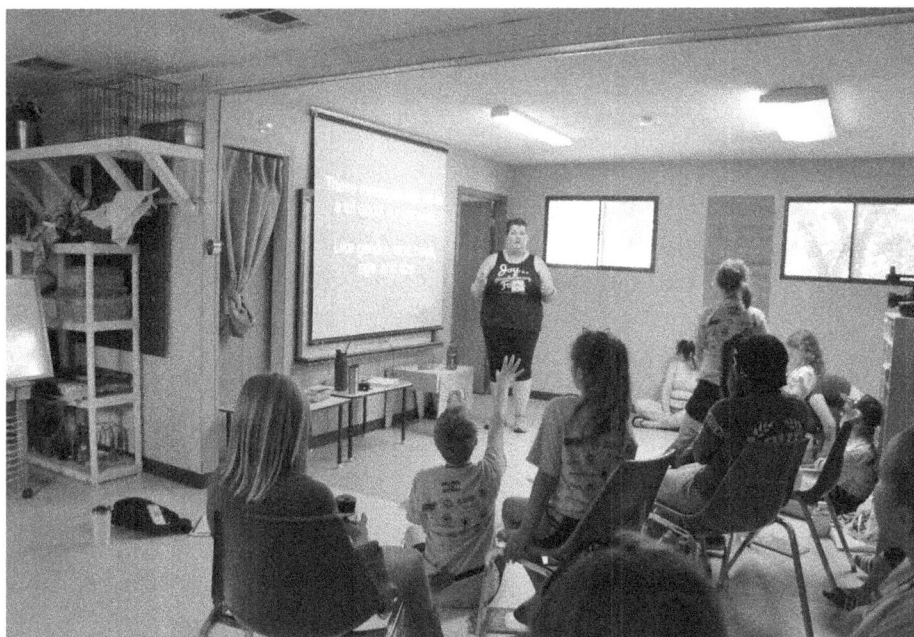

Figure 1. The author leads a media literacy workshop at Girls Rock Camp.

I assess the skepticism that fills the room.

"I'm serious." I assert. "Anyone can wear a crop top. Anyone can put a crop top on their body." I wait for the giggles to die down before I continue. "For real, there is no wrong way to have a body."

I did not anticipate this conversational turn, but, in the moment, nothing is more important than conveying this point.

"Repeat after me," I instruct them, "There is no wrong way to have a body."

"There is no wrong way to have a body," they echo.

"Again. There is no wrong way to have a body!" I am fully animated now.

It starts slowly, but the chanting builds – louder and louder until a chorus of "THERE IS NO WRONG WAY TO HAVE A BODY!" fills the small classroom.

These are important conversations to have with kids. After all, it's difficult to believe that "there is no wrong way to have a body" when the whole world is telling them otherwise. Research shows that young people are inundated with negative media messages about their bodies (Martin 2010). So much, in fact, that by six-years-old young girls start to express concerns about their body weight and size (Smolak 2011). By the time they reach elementary school, 40% of girls ages six to twelve-years-old are concerned about becoming "too fat" or "too big" (Smolak 2011).

In an effort to confront critical body image among kids, health care professionals encourage adults to teach kids about "body positivity" (Hayes

2018; Kroon Van Diest 2018). According to pediatric psychologist, Ashley Kroon Van Diest (2018), teaching kids different ways to be "positive" about their bodies helps decrease bullying, protects against negative self-image, and prevents kids from changing their body weight in unhealthy ways.

Despite the potential benefits, few kids' camps and organizations tackle body positivity in either philosophy or practice. While researchers report that kids might be engaging with a social justice curriculum outside of the home (Bartell 2013; Darling-Hammond, French, and Garcia-Lopez 2002; Gutstein 2006; Nygreen 2013), none discuss how youth organizations might be implementing body positive programming for kids.

Girls Rock Camp is an exception. On the surface, Girls Rock Camp is a kids' summer program where participants learn instruments, form bands, and write songs. Although make no mistake, Girls Rock Camp is a political project. This radical, youth-centered organization encourages girls and gender-nonconforming kids to get loud, make noise, and take up space. Girls Rock Camp prides itself as a pro-feminist, body positive space where kids and adults are free to express themselves regardless of size or ability.

In this study, I highlight the importance of kids' resistance work, with special attention to kid-led body positivity at Girls Rock Camp. Using this site as a case study, I ask the following research questions: 1) How do adult volunteers and youth campers work to make Girls Rock Camp a body positive space? 2) In what ways do kids resist oppressive beauty and body norms? And, finally, 3) Does fat stigma still persist in body positive spaces? Pulling from my own experiences as a (fat) camp counselor, I utilize over 45-hours of participant observation in order to answer these questions. This research emphasizes the unequal work that kids – and fat people – must do in order to make body positive spaces more inclusive. Furthermore, this project highlights the important role of youth activism in fat acceptance while also exposing the constraints that make body positivity difficult to achieve, even in a feminist, activist-oriented organization.

Literature review

Body positivity is in vogue. Born from the early Fat Liberation Movement, body positivity was originally lauded as the cure-all for discriminatory practices against marginalized bodies (Cooper 2016; Mull 2018). Designed to celebrate bodies that did not fit hegemonic beauty standards, body positivity became a subversive tactic used to defy cultural messages that suggest fat, queer, Black, brown, or disabled bodies are socially undesirable (Mull 2018). This, however, is no longer the case. Contemporary fat activists assert that body positivity was co-opted by capitalist endeavors (Dionne 2017; West 2018). Now, as feminist writer, Evette Dionne (2017) argues, capitalism has warped body positivity into "selling, not protecting, marginalized bodies" (p. 1).

Specifically, contemporary (or, rather, co-opted) body positivity does little to address fat stigma and discrimination. After all, "body" positive does not necessarily mean "fat" positive. Fatphobia continues to permeate through body positive culture and spaces. For example, many young girls and women engage in "fat talk" as a form of emotional labor (Gruys 2012; Nichter 2001). Fat talk works to validate people while simultaneously disassociating them from fatness. This often sounds like, "You're not fat, you're perfect!" By othering fat folks as the antithesis of desire, fat talk perpetuates a culture of fatphobia and discrimination. This creates an unequal hierarchy that privileges thin bodies and punishes fatness. Pro-fat feminists lament that true and radical body positivity is not possible in cultures that continue to shame fat bodies (Rutter 2017). True body positivity works to protect marginalized bodies from discrimination and oppression. Evette Dionne (2017) captures this sentiment when she writes: "If it's not about upending the dieting industry or protecting fat, trans, and disabled people from discrimination, it's not body positive" (p. 1).

Another problem with contemporary body positivity is that it asserts that people, especially women, are responsible for loving themselves unconditionally. Although seemingly innocuous, many feminist critics say that this brand of body positivity is just another way to victim blame marginalized communities. According to feminist writer, Amanda Mull (2018), "Contemporary body positivity makes it incumbent on people with non-conforming bodies to change their own self-perception without requiring anyone with any power to question what created the phenomenon in the first place" (p. 1). Instead of challenging macro institutions that dehumanize noncompliant bodies, this brand of body positivity shames women for their internalized insecurity. Nowadays, body positive movements erase systemic responsibility. Instead, they dictate how marginalized people should relate to their own bodies.

Contemporary body positivity also suppresses expressions of body dissatisfaction. Scholars note that corporeal insecurity is a byproduct of toxic cultural environments (Thompson and Stice 2001; Kilbourne 2000; MacNevin 2003; McDonald and Thompson 1992; Pipher 1994). Yet, in this model of "self-love," insecurity is considered a personal failure. Critics point to these pressures in body positive spaces. Adherents are expected to present themselves as pro-body all the time (Mull 2018; Rutter 2017). Not only does this silence dissent, but it also suggests that there is a "right" way to engage with our bodies. Feminist scholar, Susan Bordo (1993, 1999), discusses this phenomenon when she writes about the contradictory "double bind." According to Bordo (1999), on one hand, society "encourages women to see themselves as defective; on the other hand, it chastises them for their insecurities" (p. 250). Unable to win, women are forced to experience both the insecurity and the shame of body positive propaganda.

Regardless of its potential shortcomings, parents and pediatricians continue to push for a "body positive" culture for kids and young adults. As youth organizations start to implement body positive curriculum for kids, the question remains: how do we see kids and adults make these spaces move inclusive? And, furthermore, do contemporary models of body positivity translate into fat acceptance and inclusion in these spaces?

Girls Rock Camp

In many ways, Girls Rock Camp is an enclave of resistance. Kids, ages eight through sixteen, work closely with adult volunteers and other kids to form their own rock band. They take up the guitar, drums, keys, or bass for the first time, start a band, write an original song, and, at the end of the week, perform their song live for family, friends, and local community members at a Girls Rock Showcase. According to their website, Girls Rock Camp is "a youth-centered music organization that cultivates an empowering space for girls, women, trans, and gender non-conforming people to collaborate and experiment in music, expression, performance, and collective care" (Girls Rock Carbondale 2017).

But unlike other summer camps, Girls Rock engages a political praxis. It incorporates a social justice curriculum revolving around workshops that teach self-defense and zine making, confronts racial, gender, and class privileges, defines and identifies consent, and teaches media literacy. Built on tenets of implicit feminism (Gifford 2011), Girls Rock prides itself as a political, action-oriented organization that serves local and global communities.

At the international level, the Girls Rock Camp Alliance claims that it "strive(s) to shift leadership towards our membership, people of color – particularly black and indigenous people, trans and gender non-conforming folks, people with disabilities, neuro-diverse people, poor and working-class people, queer folks, femmes and feminine people, fat people and people of size, and people outside the U.S. and the West" (Girls Rock Camp Alliance 2018). In order to challenge systematic oppression, Girls Rock actively incorporates marginalized voices at the top levels of their leadership. Then, from the top down, it works to make space for folks who are politically and socially disenfranchised. This is no small feat for a kids' summer camp. However, Girls Rock is an ambitious program that aims to create safe spaces where both campers and volunteers can express themselves regardless of ability or size.

Methods

I utilize participant observation to analyze interactions among youth campers and adult volunteers at Girls Rock Camp. In the summer of 2018, I spent nine hours a day for five consecutive days at Girls Rock Camp. Before camp started, I gained written permission from the camp director to be a participant observer in this space. My researcher status was well-known among all of the camp volunteers. I was also open with campers about my role as 1) a social researcher, and 2) a mandated reporter. Ethically, it was important for me to be forthright with everyone at camp. While most campers were initially curious about my "school project," many of them quickly forgot about it and treated me like an ordinary camp counselor.

I consistently wore a backpack at camp. This is where I kept all of my research tools. I made sure to carry a notebook with lots of pens – along with my essential water bottle, earplugs, and camp bandana. Whenever I witnessed an interesting conversation or interaction, I would pull out my notebook and jot down a quick note in order to remind myself about it later. I took numerous field notes in my research journal, cataloging "magnified moments" (Messner 2000, 766) that resisted, or, perhaps, reproduced fat stigma and discrimination in this site. Later, once at home, I elaborated on my initial notes. I would often journal for up to an hour every night after camp. This was an opportunity for me to think critically about the day's events and to organize my thoughts and observations. After camp week was over, I started to code my research journal. I looked for recurring themes and patterns that might illustrate how campers engaged in body positive resistance work, and what this activism might mean for fat folks at camp.

Although research was my primary goal, I also served as a camp counselor in this space. I occupied both of these roles – that of researcher and counselor – simultaneously. As a counselor, my main responsibilities were to make sure that campers were physically safe, hydrated, and emotionally content. This was no small task. After all, it is difficult to manage thirty-five rockstars who are constantly misplacing their water bottles. In spite of these challenges, I provided emotional support, boundless enthusiasm, and served as a willing participant during spontaneous dance parties. It was also important to be there for instrumental tasks. During camp, it was my duty to escort campers to and from music instruction, remind them to clean up after themselves, and make sure that everyone wore their earplugs during band practice.

Counseling also provided a unique vantage point at camp. As a camp counselor, I was privy to both frontstage and backstage operations (Goffman 1959). I followed my band to social justice workshops, listened to them collaborate during band practice, and helped them design an original band logo during the merchandising workshop. This access allowed me to get closer with campers and fellow volunteers. I was, after all, an insider at camp. I developed emotional relationships with many of the people in this space. Although everyone was aware of my researcher status, many of them opened up to me as a friend or mentor.

I was also an emotional caretaker at camp. In addition to my role as a camp counselor, I served as a volunteer coordinator. It was my responsibility to vet potential volunteers, manage camp scheduling, and address adult participants' needs or concerns. Typically, this meant that I resolved the occasional scheduling mishap. Other times, however, I would lend a listening ear or shoulder to cry on. I mediated interpersonal volunteer conflicts, consoled campers (and some counselors) during emotional meltdowns, and reminded everyone that they were doing a great job.

Not only was this role emotionally taxing, but it was also physical. As a fat, white, cisgender woman, several of my identities (both visible and invisible) shaped my experiences at camp. All of my interactions – with campers, parents, and volunteers – were processed through a lens of fat visibility. Embodying white femme fatness provided a unique perspective while at camp. Operating as a fat body, there, at camp, allowed me to occupy a critical in-between: both as a social researcher and marginalized body. My observations, as a fat researcher, work to expose the constraints that make body positivity difficult to achieve, even in a feminist, activist-oriented organization.

Findings

Below, I present my findings on how Girls Rock Camp strives to promote a body positive culture for both kids and adults. I argue that campers actively challenge fat stigma and hegemonic beauty norms. They show their stomachs, write anti-shame lyrics, and create zines that showcase diverse beauty and body types. However, echoes of fatphobia are still present at camp. For instance, campers draw on fat stigma to police other kids for what, and how much, they eat at lunch. Campers, as well as adult volunteers, engage in validating fat talk to let others know that "they aren't fat, they're beautiful!" And, finally, adult volunteers and campers encounter (and struggle with) pressures to model body positivity in this space. While Girls Rock Camp indeed helps kids fight against oppressive body norms, it simultaneously privileges thin adult bodies at an organizational level.

Policing bodies

The cafeteria is crowded. Campers and counselors fill the long, picnic-style lunch tables. Kids as young as eight-years-old run around the outer hallways while the older campers, at a cool sixteen years, converse on tabletops. One camper, sporting a fresh electric-blue hairdo, taps a drumstick against the cafeteria wall. Tap..tap..tap-tap-tap..tap.

Exiting the food line with a slice of pizza, I make my way into the lunch room. My eyes scan the room as I look for a seat big enough to accommodate my body. I'm still searching for a spot when I notice a small camper re-enter the food line for seconds. There is always plenty of food at camp and it is not unusual for folks to go back for seconds – or even thirds.

"Whoa!" I hear someone exclaim as she makes her way back to the table. "How many slices have you had?" a fellow camper asks her.

"Three," she grins as she starts to devour her fourth slice of pepperoni pizza.

"That's what I thought," her friend chides. "You better watch out or you're gonna get fat!" Both laugh as they continue to eat lunch.

Young campers police food consumption regularly at Girls Rock Camp. After all, they warn, the penalty for overeating is fatness. Although Girls Rock actively claims to be a "body positive" space, there are several instances where campers make anti-fat statements. Encouraged by camp staff to challenge hegemonic beauty standards, campers can easily criticize media messages surrounding size at workshops and through song writing. These conversations, however, revolve around unrealistic pressures to be thin. Campers never broach the subject of fat acceptance or celebration. Fatness is the borderland. While campers expressed frustrations with cultural fixations on thinness, no one was willing to embrace the alternative. For example, one camper exclaimed, "I don't think dieting is very healthy. Like, no one is supposed to be as thin as these models." Pushing back against heterofeminine size standards that keep women small, campers agree that you shouldn't have to lose weight to be socially acceptable. Fatness, on the other hand, is still an undesirable physical state. Body positivity, as practiced at camp, is a static phenomenon. Accepting your body – in its current state – is OK. Change, especially in the context of weight gain or loss, however, is met with peer policing (Figure 2).

Campers are especially anxious about fat stigma. Although many of them speak out against peer bullying and discrimination, no one wanted to be the fat kid at camp. After all, fat youth experience increased levels of social harassment and violence (Hayden-Wade et al. 2005; Latner and Stunkard 2003; Puhl and Latner 2007; Weinstock and Krehbiel 2009). And, while I never directly observed weight-related bullying at camp, size-policing comments imply that it wasn't an impossibility.

In an interesting twist, campers actively resisted the idea that they should have to appeal to anyone else's idea of beauty. Specifically, in an original camp song, campers write:

"Hiding in a violent storm
No one wants to see my form
I don't wanna care what people think
My thoughts should only matter to me
I just wanna be free."

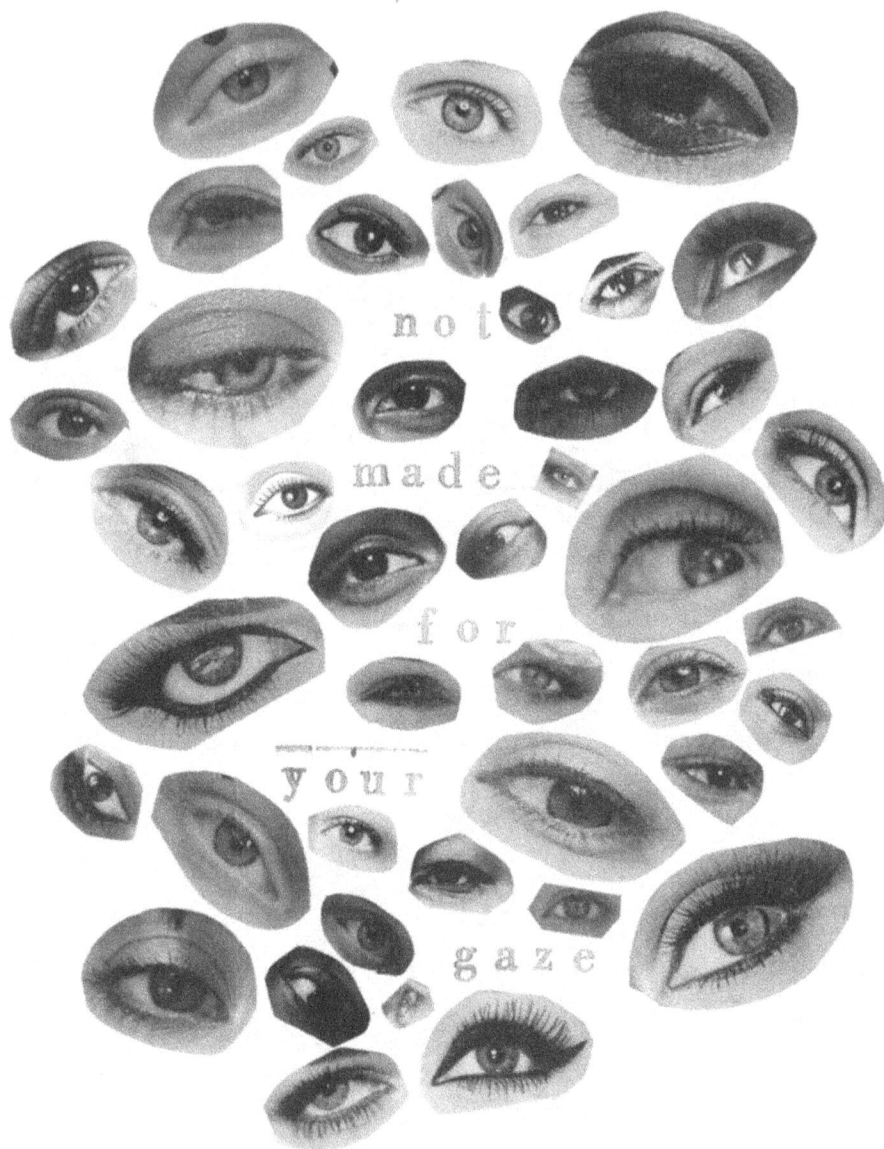

Figure 2. Camper's original zine page that challenges societal pressures and censure.

This song suggests that campers don't want to care about what others think about their "form." Instead, they want to be "free" from social expectations and body policing. Even as kids speak out to disrupt mainstream narratives about societal pressure, they are harassed for eating too much pizza at lunchtime. Echoing Rutter's (2017) findings, interactions at Girls Rock Camp demonstrate that contemporary body positivity does little to combat fat stigma in youth culture. Fatphobia continues to permeate through body positive culture and spaces – even in a feminist, activist-oriented organization.

Structural barriers also work to police adult bodies at camp. Specifically, the biggest challenge for counselors of size was fitting into the long, picnic-style tables in the cafeteria. Campers and counselors ate both breakfast and lunch at these tables every day. These tables, however, were not accommodating for everybody at camp. Fat and/or disabled participants were barred from group participation in the cafeteria. I experienced this first-hand while at camp. As one of the only fat women there, I frequently found that mealtime was an isolating experience. After all, accepting a camper's sitting invitation at lunch meant having to squeeze my size-28 frame into bench-style cafeteria seating.

"Come and sit with us," campers would exclaim. "We saved you a seat!"

"For sure," I lied. "I just have to go and do something first."

I used this excuse, almost daily at camp, right before I sneaked off to the volunteer breakroom. Unwilling to explain how I could not fit, and without an available alternative, I excused myself from group activities in the cafeteria.

This exclusion was a sizeist oversight. Structural barriers, like seating accommodations, police whose bodies can, and cannot, be included at tables of power (or breakfast foods). Unable to access a seat, I was rendered invisible to both campers and counselors during lunchtime. This was problematic in many ways. Specifically, this suggests that body positivity does not necessarily mean fat accessibility or inclusivity. Despite their attempts to cultivate a body positive environment for "everybody," Girls Rock Camp obviously falls short. This program, as organized by thin, standard-size adults, upholds thin and able-bodied privilege at the organizational level. Despite the resistance work that kids are doing at the interpersonal-level, Girls Rock Camp continues to police fat bodies' access to power and space. This reproduces the shame and stigma associated with being fat in the social world.

"Reassuring" fat talk

Back at the media literacy workshop, I pass out a stack of glossy beauty magazines. Campers share the magazines among themselves, taking one from the pile before they pass the rest around.

"Here, I want you to look through these magazines. Do you see yourself represented in any of them?" I ask the group of campers sitting around me.

I watch as they flip through dog-eared issues of *Cosmopolitan*, *Vogue*, and *InStyle*. I notice that a few of them start to shake their heads "no," eyebrows furrowed, expressions serious.

"Who don't we see?" I probe.

"Black people, or really, anyone who isn't white," answers an older camper.

"I don't see anyone with zits! Like, their skin is always perfect," another preteen laments.

Another girl raises her hand, slowly, and waits on me to call on her.

"They're all really skinny. I'm not like that," she says quietly.

"You're all right," I nod. "Not everyone is represented in these pictures. In fact, none of these people are fat like me." I feel their eyes travel the length of my full-sized body, assessing the weighted curve of my thighs, waist, and chest. "The closest representation of my body is probably the 'before' picture in a weight loss ad."

I hear a few sharp inhales and I watch as they shift uncomfortably in their seats. My body occupies space, like the metaphorical elephant in the room. Unsightly, and, therefore not seen. Or, at least, not mentioned. After all, it is not polite to point out the obvious. I feel other campers pick up on the shared tension.

One of them breaks: "You're not fat! You're beautiful!" a young camper exclaims.

I pause. *But why can't I be both?*

While at camp, campers expressed affection for me in a lot of ways. They chatted with me during free time, they were excited to share their snacks, and several of them gifted me with original artwork and band buttons. At the workshop, however, campers revert to fat talk in order to reassure me that I am "beautiful." By resorting to fat talk, campers assume that I do not want to be fat. In their attempt to disassociate me from fatness, kids reinforce the notion that beauty cannot coincide with physical fatness. Refusing to categorize me as a transgressive (or bad) social body, they expose internalized fatphobia. This demonstrates how care work is constructed to erase fat identities while simultaneously privileging hegemonic heterofemininity.

Even though campers encourage women to "break the norms" in original zine art (Figure 3), they are unable to endorse identities that challenge thin beauty standards. In this instance, I feel responsible to remind youth campers that fat identities (and bodies) are OK. I argue that this – resisting fat talk in social situations – is another form of emotional labor. By carefully challenging the youth, I actively (and unequally) work to disrupt hegemonic norms that privilege thin bodies as exclusively beautiful. This demonstrates how Girls Rock unintentionally privileges thin bodies at an organizational level. Fat people must do unequal work in order to make body positive spaces more inclusive. This is yet another way in which fat bodies are expected to appeal for equal consideration in a world that discriminates against them.

Fat talk was not exclusive to my relationship with campers. My body frequently held tension as other volunteers reaffirmed their size privilege through self-deprecating fat talk. Adult volunteers also used fat talk to reassure me that I wasn't "too fat" or "that big" at camp. Specifically, this occurred during a do-it-yourself screen-printing workshop. After designing an original band logo, campers (and their counselors) get to print their design on a camp t-shirt using ink, screens, and squeegees.

After our band finished screen-printing, we hung our t-shirts to dry with the others on a wooden clothes rack. Unlike my campers, however, I forgot

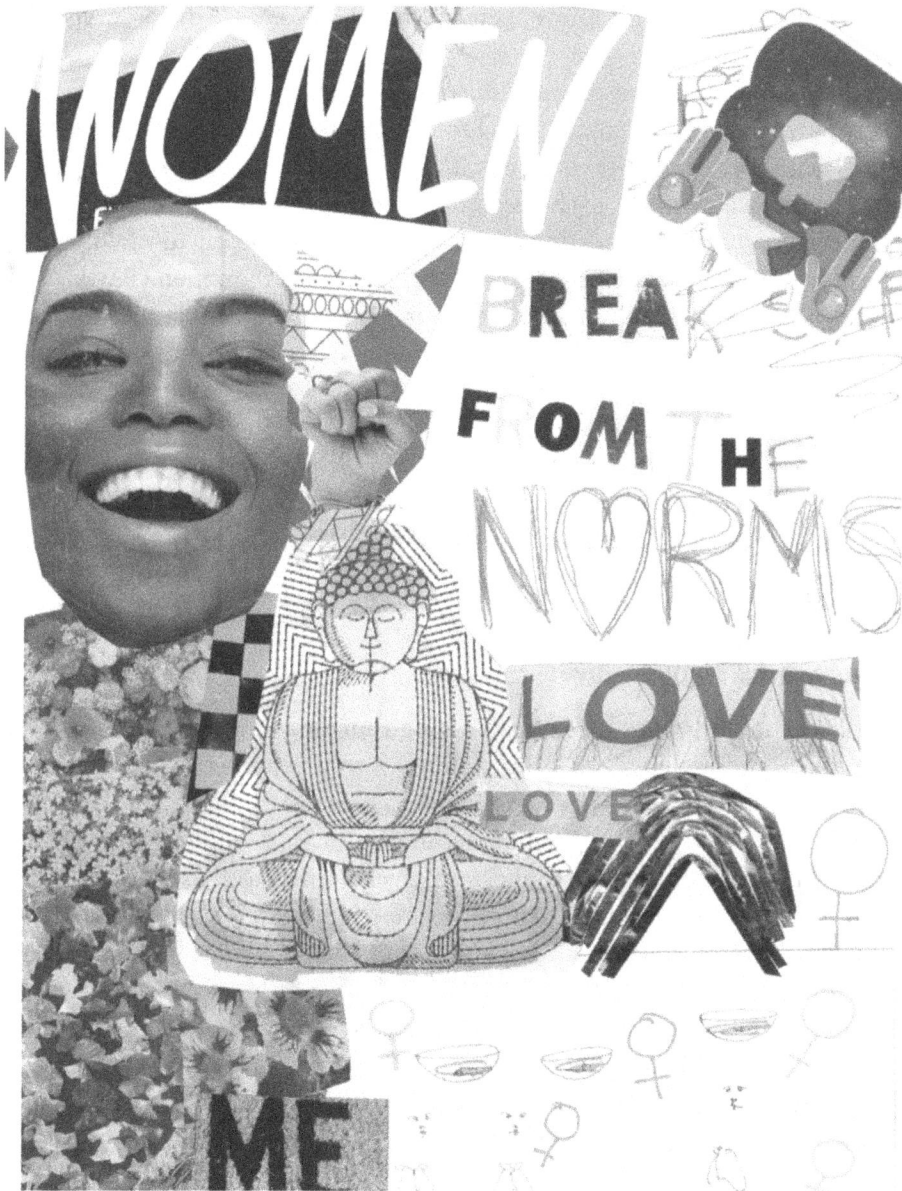

Figure 3. Camper's original zine page that encourages women to "break from the norms".

to write my name on the t-shirt tag. Brie, a first-time camp counselor, was quick to catch my mistake.

"Umm, someone forgot to write their name inside their shirt," she informed us as we waited for our shirts to dry. I instantly realized that I was the culprit.

"Oh, it's mine. I'm sorry," I offered. "None of my campers wear a 3X."

I watched my joke fall flat as her face flushed with color.

"Well, I mean, I didn't know," she stuttered. "Besides," she assured, "You don't look that big."

Brie uses fat talk to reassure me that I don't "look" as big as my actual size. Specifically, she uses fat talk as a tool to disembody me from my transgressive fatness. This device, as Brie employs it, is supposed to reassure me that I am still attractive according to heterofeminine measures. Her reaction recalls previous research that finds that women are not supposed to be "that big," but are meant to be smaller and to take up less space than men (Bartky 1988; Bordo 1990, 1993; Chernin 1981; Mazur 1986). Brie's exclamation, that I don't look "that big," is a coded compliment. After all, if Brie admits that I am too large – or worse, fat – I could be socially undesirable (Bordo 1993; Braziel and LeBesco 2001; Braziel 2001; Mull 2018; Popenoe 2005). Although Girls Rock Camp claims to be an accepting place for "fat people and people of size," reoccurring fat talk exposes internalized fatphobia (Girls Rock Camp Alliance 2018). This illustrates how kids, and fat folks, do unequal work to make spaces more size inclusive.

Pressure to be body positive

I'm excited to go to lunch. It's been a long morning at camp and I am ready to sit down and recharge. As I am walking into the cafeteria, however, Dani, a fellow camp counselor, stops me.

"Hey, can I talk to you about something?"

It is the fourth day of camp and I am accustomed to these conversational starters. As a camp organizer, I am routinely approached with other volunteers' problems or concerns.

"Of course! What's up?"

"I mean, umm, can I talk with you privately?" For the first time, I notice that her eyes are brimming with tears.

"How can I help?" I start cautiously, as I walk with her to the outside playground. I'm not sure where this is headed. We both take a seat at a shaded picnic table.

"Like, I get it. I know we are supposed to be all 'body positive' here. But, I can't be. I've gained 20 pounds this past year and I feel it. Everywhere. I don't know who I am. I don't know how to deal with it." Her words come faster as tears stream down her face.

I freeze.

"What am I supposed to do?" She asks me.

Dani relays that she is "supposed" to feel good about her body at Girls Rock Camp. Citing pressure to be "all body positive" in this space, she addresses a fundamental concern about contemporary body positivity movements: is radical self-love just another performance piece? Are socially marginalized people expected to "perform" body positivity in the service of others? The pressure to be body positive in this feminist space conflicts with (and suppresses) Dani's feelings about her body. She views her insecurity as a personal failure. Dani is experiencing a double bind – as she feels both defective about gaining weight *and* insecure about her poor body image (Bordo 1993, 1999). Instead of examining external conditions that fuel internalized fatphobia, Dani attaches herself to the idea that she is doing body positivity poorly. After all, mainstream body positivity movements demand that noncompliant bodies uphold societal pretense at all cost. This echoes Rutter's (2017) findings about self-expression and the body positive movement. Social displays of body positivity do little to address fat stigma in its contemporary form. My interaction with Dani suggests that fatphobia remains present in this space. It is a persistent constraint that makes body positivity difficult to achieve, even in a feminist, activist-oriented organization (Figure 4).

I, too, experienced pressure to be body positive at camp. Specifically, I felt the pressure to model hyper-positivity about my fat body. Fatphobia and stigma make it difficult to live in the "real world" (Bordo 1993; Braziel 2001; Braziel and LeBesco 2001; Mull 2018; Popenoe 2005). Therefore, at camp, I

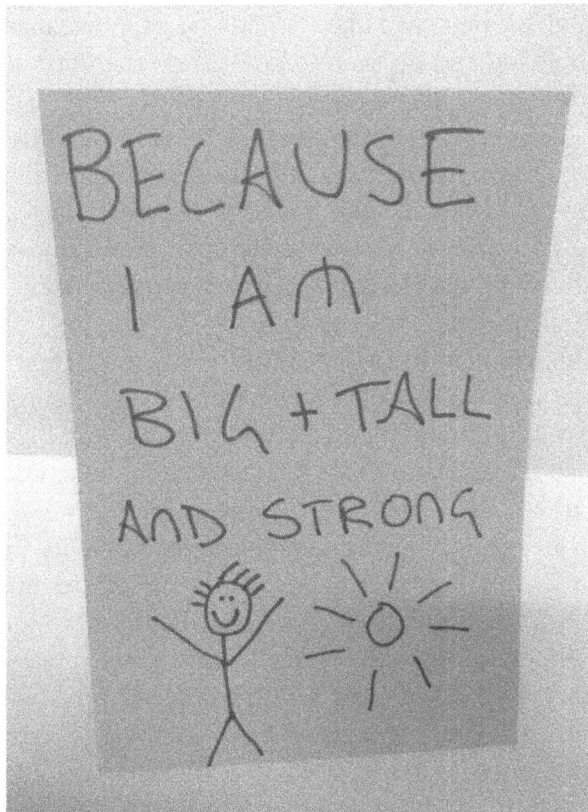

Figure 4. A camper cites size and strength as a reason why they rock.

worked unequally hard to make sure that fat bodies were welcome and celebrated. In order to do this, I actively challenged implicit fatphobia from campers, adult volunteers, and even parents.

This happened on the first day of camp. While I stood at the front door, welcoming the arriving parents and campers, a camper's mother carefully approached me before registering her daughter.

"Hi, uh, I'm Allie's mom," she started.

"It's nice to meet you," I replied, smiling brightly at her young, round-faced kid. "We're going to have a great time this week!"

"Uh, listen," the mom continued as her daughter joined the other kids in the morning assembly room. "This is Allie's first time at camp, and I'm worried that she won't make any friends. You don't think the other kids are going to make fun of her, right? Because she's, uh, bigger?"

I raised my eyebrows and lowered my voice, "Absolutely not," I reassured her. "We work really hard to make sure everyone has a good time at camp. Although I can keep an eye out if that makes you feel better."

"Yes, please. I'm sure this seems silly," she broached, "But I knew *you* could understand."

This interaction is embedded with social meaning. First, Allie's mom is scared that her plus-size daughter won't be able to make any friends. This is not unfounded given that fat kids, and adults, experience higher levels of weight-related bullying and discrimination. However, Allie's mom continues to insinuate that I can relate to weight-related bullying. This assumption suggests that Allie's mom 1) reads me as a fat body in this space, and 2) expects that I, too, have experienced size discrimination. Allie's mom relays her suspicions in coded fat talk. She will not openly acknowledge my fatness; but expects me to "understand" her daughter's predicament. Allie's mom expects me to do more work (as a fat body at camp) in order to protect her daughter from bullies.

Not only do parents expect me to do more work for their fat kids, but I feel this pressure as well. Allie's welfare becomes my personal undertaking. Being a fellow fat person (and, perhaps, adult role model), I am compelled to behave in a hyper-positive way about my own fatness. Like Dani, I know that I am supposed to be "all body positive" while at camp. In this case, however, I feel an added pressure to specifically model fat positivity and acceptance. This illustrates the emotional care and labor that fat bodies must do in order to make body positive spaces, like Girls Rock Camp, more inclusive.

There was, however, kid-led resistance to these pressures at camp. Although both adult volunteers and youth campers expressed anxiety about doing body confidence or mentorship the "right way," campers chose to actively speak out against its effects. Specifically, campers address the pressure to engage in false personas while writing the original song, "Let Me Be

Free." According to the lyrics, campers are distressed about the need to falsely present authenticity to other people. They sing:

"Feeling oppressed, I'm upset
Ashamed to show who I am
And they wanna tell us to be ourselves
I feel like this is all a scam
I just wanna be me."

Campers imply that "they," or, others in society, tell them that they should just be themselves. The youth disclose, however, that they feel "ashamed" to show their true selves. This leads to feelings of oppression and disconnect. Calling it all a "scam," campers actively resist the notion that there is a standard model for self-expression. Echoing Mull's (2018) own assessment of body positivity, the campers assert that "others" are not sincere when they tell youth to "be themselves." Kids, and, by extension, marginalized bodies, are only allowed to be themselves when their identities align with socially acceptable norms. This, however, is not true expression or freedom. Campers call out all systems of oppression that shame marginalized identities and claim that they, "just wanna be me."

This piece demonstrates the work that young people do to resist hegemonic norms and discriminatory practices. Campers claim that they want to be free from social systems that tell them how they should feel about their bodies and identities. This critique challenges macro institutions that dehumanize noncompliant bodies and identities. It illustrates the important work that kids are doing in order to change social scripts about privilege, marginalized identities, and oppression.

Conclusion

The daily merch workshop is about to start. This is where campers get hands-on experience with do-it-yourself merchandise design and creation. Half of my band members are designing buttons to sell at the showcase, while others are decorating old denim patches with puffy paint (Figure 5).

"Hey, what's up?" I greet a table of campers as I take an empty seat next to them.

"Does anyone want to finish screen printing our band logo?" I suggest before I notice a camper holding a pair of scissors to the hem of her band t-shirt. Without preamble, she cuts a jagged line across the bottom of her cotton shirt.

"There," she exclaims. "Now it's a crop top!"

"Cool!" Another camper chimes in. "I want a crop top, too!"

I watch as multiple kids start cutting off their t-shirt bottoms. Some of their lines are steady and smooth, others are a bit rougher – asymmetrical edges that are beginning to curl upward – exposing soft, round bellies.

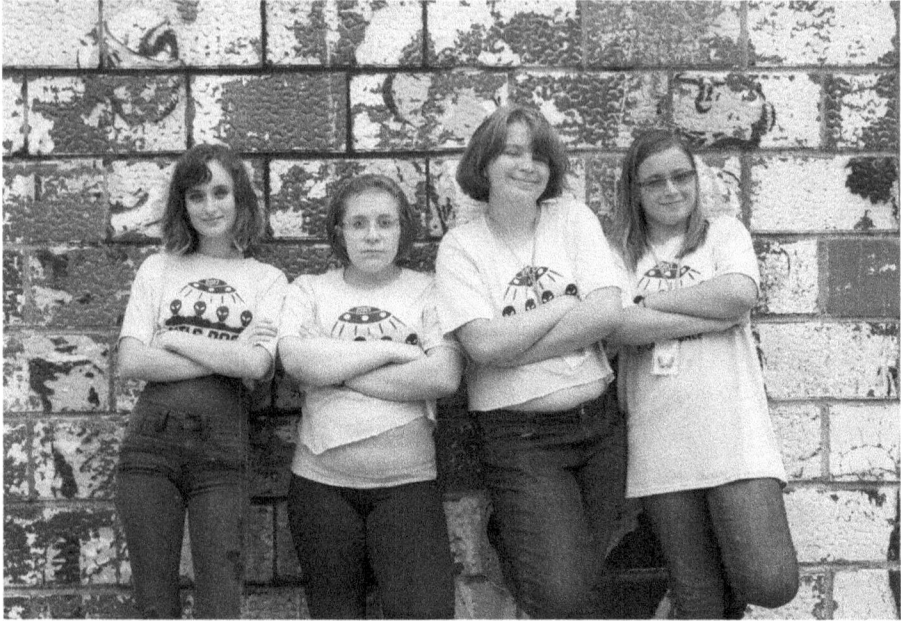

Figure 5. Campers pose with self-made crop tops for their band photos.

One of my band members grins at me as she tugs her new shirt over her head.

"Anybody can wear a crop top!" She beams. "What do you think?"

Resistance narratives are complicated stories that demonstrate the constraints and contradictions that make change difficult to achieve (Hollander and Einwohner 2004). This, I argue, is the case at Girls Rock Camp. Campers draw on fat stigma to police kids for what, and how much, they eat. Kids, as well as adult volunteers, engage in validating fat talk to let others know that they are valued. And, finally, adults and kids encounter (and struggle with) pressures to model body positivity while at camp. Using Girls Rock Camp as a case study, I argue that body positivity is not enough. Fat activists must work harder to ensure that spaces (even radical kids' camps) are inclusive and welcoming towards fat folks. Although part of the picture, this is not the complete story. Kids and adults still do important resistance work in these spaces. Specifically, kids challenge size discrimination on an interpersonal level by cropping t-shirts, performing anti-shame songs, and questioning unrealistic beauty standards. Adults also work to support youth activism in a movement that "amplifies voices that have otherwise been told to be silent" (Girls Rock Camp Alliance 2018). Together they attempt to build an inclusive world where, truly, there is no wrong way to have a body. In an effort to highlight the importance of their fat activism, this project works to expose the constraints that make body positivity difficult to achieve, while celebrating the hard-won battles that they accomplish.

Disclosure statement

No potential conflict of interest was reported by the author.

References

Bartell, Tonya Gau. 2013. "Learning to Teach Mathematics for Social Justice: Negotiating Social Justice and Mathematical Goals." *Journal for Research in Mathematical Education* 44 (1):129–63.

Bartky, S. L. 1988. ""Foucault, Femininity, and the Modernization of Patriarchal Power." In *The Politics of Women's Bodies: Sexuality, Appearance, and Behavior*, edited by R. Weitz. New York, NY: Oxford University Press.

Bordo, Susan. 1990. "Material Girl: The Effacements of Postmodern Culture." *Michigan Quarterly Review* 29:653–77.

Bordo, Susan. 1993. *Unbearable Weight: Feminism, Western Culture, and the Body*. Berkeley: University of California Press.

Bordo, Susan. 1999. "Feminism, Foucault, and the Politics of the Body." In *Feminist Theory and the Body: A Reader*, edited by Janet Price and Margrit Shildrick, 246–57. New York, NY: Routledge.

Braziel, Jana Evans. 2001. "Sex and Fat Chics: Deterritorializing the Fat Female Body." In *Bodies Out of Bounds: Fatness and Transgression*, edited by J. E. Braziel and K. LeBesco, 231–56. Berkeley: University of California Press.

Braziel, Jana Evans, and Kathleen LeBesco, eds. 2001. *Bodies Out of Bounds: Fatness and Transgression*. Berkeley: University of California Press.

Chernin, Kim. 1981. *The Obsession: Reflections on the Tyranny of Slenderness*. New York, NY: Harper & Row.

Cooper, Charlotte. 2016. *Fat Activism: A Radical Social Movement*. Bristol: HammerOn Press.

Darling-Hammond, Linda, Jennifer C. French, and Silvia Paloma Garcia-Lopez. 2002. *Learning to Teach for Social Justice*. New York, NY: Teachers College Press.

Dionne, Evette. 2017. "The Fragility of Body Positivity: How a Radical Movement Lost Its Way." Retrieved February 2, 2019 (https://www.bitchmedia.org/article/fragility-body-positivity).

Gifford, Danielle. 2011. "Show or Tell? Feminist Dilemmas and Implicit Feminism at Girls' Rock Camp." *Gender & Society* 25 (5):569–88. doi:10.1177/0891243211415978

Girls Rock Camp Alliance. 2018. "Points of Unity." Retrieved July 10, 2018 (https://www.girlsrockcampalliance.org/about).

Girls Rock Carbondale. 2017. "Girls Rock Carbondale." Retrieved July 10, 2018 (http://www.girlsrockcarbondale.com).

Goffman, Erving. 1959. *The Presentation of Self in Everyday Life*. Garden City, NY: Double Day Anchor Books.

Gruys, Kjerstin. 2012. "Does This Make Me Look Fat? Aesthetic Labor and Fat Talk as Emotional Labor in a Women's Plus-Size Clothing Store." *Social Problems* 59 (4):481–500. doi:10.1525/sp.2012.59.4.481

Gutstein, Eric. 2006. *Reading and Writing the World with Mathematics: Toward a Pedagogy for Social Justice*. New York, NY: Routledge.

Hayden-Wade, H. A., R. I. Stein, A. Ghaderi, B. E. Saelens, M. F. Zabinski, and D. E. Wilfley. 2005. "Prevalence, Characteristics, and Correlates of Teasing Experiences among Overweight Children Vs. Non-Overweight Peers." *Obesity Research* 13: 1381–92. doi: 10.1038/oby.2005.167.

Hayes, Dayle. 2018. "5 Ways to Promote a Positive Body Image for Kids." Retrieved February 2, 2019 (https://www.eatright.org/health/weight-loss/your-health-and-your-weight/5-ways-to-promote-a-positive-body-image-for-kids).

Hollander, Jocelyn A., and Rachel L. Einwohner. 2004. "Conceptualizing Resistance." *Sociological Forum* 19 (4):533–54. doi:10.1007/s11206-004-0694-5

Kevin, Thompson, J., and Eric Stice. 2001. "Thin Ideal Internalization: Mounting Evidence for a New Risk Factor for Body Image Disturbance and Eating Pathology." *Current Directions in Psychological Science* 10 (5):181–83. doi:10.1111/1467-8721.00144

Kilbourne, Jean. 2000. *Can't Buy My Love: How Advertising Changes the Way We Think and Feel*. New York, NY: Free Press.

Kroon Van Diest, Ashley. 2018. "Body Positivity: An Important Message for Girls, AND Boys." Retrieved February 2, 2019 (https://www.nationwidechildrens.org/family-resources-education/700childrens/2018/10/body-positivity).

Latner, Janet D., and Albert J. Stunkard. 2003. "Getting Worse: The Stigmatization of Obese Children." *Obesity Research* 11: 452–56. doi: 10.1038/oby.2003.61.

MacNevin, Audrey. 2003. "Exercising Options: Holistic Health and Technical Beauty in Gendered Accounts of Bodywork." *The Sociological Quarterly* 44 (2):271–89. doi:10.1111/j.1533-8525.2003.tb00558.x

Martin, J. B. 2010. "The Development of Ideal Body Image Perceptions in the United States." *Nutrition Today* 45 (3):98–100. doi:10.1097/NT.0b013e3181dec6a2

Mazur, Allan. 1986. "U.S. Trends in Feminine Beauty and Overadaptation." *The Journal of Sex Research* 22 (3):281–303. doi:10.1080/00224498609551309

McDonald, K., and K. L. Thompson. 1992. "Eating Disturbances, Body Image Dissatisfaction, and Reasons for Exercising: Gender Differences and Coorelational Findings." *International Journal of Eating Disorders* 11 (3):289–92. doi:10.1002/1098-108X(199204)11:3<289::AID-EAT2260110314>3.0.CO;2-F

Messner, Michael A. 2000. "The Barbie Girls versus the Sea Monsters: Children Constructing Gender." *Gender & Society* 14 (6):765–84. doi:10.1177/089124300014006004

Mull, Amanda. 2018. "Body Positivity Is a Scam: How a Movement Intended to Lift up Women Really Just Limits Their Acceptable Emotions. Again." Retrieved July 12, 2018 (https://www.racked.com/2018/6/5/17236212/body-positivity-scam-dove-campaign-ads).

Nichter, Mimi. 2001. *Fat Talk: What Girls and Their Parents Say about Dieting*. Cambridge, MA: Harvard University Press.

Nygreen, Kysa. 2013. *These Kids: Identity, Agency, and Social Justice at a Last Chance High School*. Chicago, IL: University of Chicago Press.

Pipher, Mary Bray. 1994. *Reviving Ophelia: Saving the Selves of Adolescent Girls*. New York, NY: Putnam.

Popenoe, Rebecca. 2005. "Ideal." In *Fat: The Anthropology of an Obsession*, edited by D. Kulick and A. Meneley, 9–28. New York, NY: Tarcher/Penguin.

Puhl, Rebecca M., and J. D. Latner. 2007. "Stigma, Obesity, and the Health of the Nation'S Children." *Psychological Bulletin* 133 (4):557–80. doi:10.1037/0033-2909.133.4.557

Rutter, Bethany. 2017. "How 'Body Positivity' Lost Its True and Radical Meaning." Retrieved July 20, 2018 (http://www.dazeddigital.com/artsandculture/article/35746/1/how-body-positivity-lost-its-true-and-radical-meaning).

Smolak, Linda. 2011. "Body Image Development in Childhood." In *Body Image: A Handbook of Science, Practice, and Prevention*, edited by T. F. Cash and L. Smolak, 67–75. New York, NY: Guilford.

Weinstock, Jacqueline, and Michelle Krehbiel. 2009. "Fat Youth as Common Targets for Bullying." In *The Fat Studies Reader*, edited by E. Rothblum and S. Solovay, 120–26. New York: New York University Press.

West, Lindy. 2018. "The Way We Talk About Bodies Has Changed. What We Do About It Comes Next." Retrieved February 2, 2019 (https://www.self.com/story/the-way-we-talk-about-bodies).

Mapping the circulation of fat hatred

Jen Rinaldi, Carla Rice, Crystal Kotow, and Emma Lind

ABSTRACT

The authors draw from affect theory and intersectionality-as-assemblage theory to conceptualize fatmisia as a complex affective force. In line with queer affect theorist Sara Ahmed's theorizing of emotion, the authors explore how fat hatred circulates as an affective economy: how it flows across, attaches to, and comes to define or value different bodies. The authors analyze interview data compiled for the research project *Through Thick & Thin* to map fat hatred circulating in healthcare contexts, on transit, and while exercising. The data yielded insight into how fat hatred obstructs access to public participation, resources, and services, by rendering public space and social exchanges uncomfortable, unwelcoming, unsafe, and inaccessible. Constellations of feelings that adhere to fat bodies become instruments of fatmisia, and operate relationally in the space between bodies with the object of erasing or expunging fat life.

We draw from affect theory and intersectionality-as-assemblage theory to conceptualize fatmisia as a complex affective force. The term *fatmisia*—the *misia* derived from the Greek *misos*, meaning hatred, dislike, or contempt—refers to hatred of fat, fatness, and fat persons. The strength of the term—and its capacity to encompass, not equate to, fatphobia or fear of fat—positions feelings about and treatment of fat persons on a register comparable to, for example, misogyny or hatred of women. Unwelcome interactions with fat persons encompass concern, judgment, dread, disdain, revulsion, and violence. These expressions share in common how they operate relationally in the spaces between bodies—how they give shape to and produce in bodies orientations, directions, and movements toward and away from other bodies. In line with queer affect theorist Sara Ahmed's (2004) theorizing of emotion, we are interested in how fat hatred circulates as an affective economy: how it flows across, attaches to, and comes to define or value different bodies.

We analyze interview data compiled for the research project *Through Thick & Thin*. For this project, we interviewed queer women and trans folk who carry a range of intersecting identity markers and express shifting locations in social relations. A majority of participants identified as being currently fat or as having been fat. They shared their experiences of how reactions that we coded under the rubric of fat hatred manifested in healthcare contexts, on transit, and while exercising. The data yielded insight into how fat hatred obstructs access to public participation, resources, and services, by rendering public space and social exchanges uncomfortable, unwelcoming, unsafe, and inaccessible. We use our data to surface the constellation of feelings that adhere to subjects, objects, and discourses, which become instruments of fatmisia, and how those instruments operate relationally in the space between bodies with the object of erasing or expunging fat life.

How fatmisia works

To make sense of hatred as affect, we turn to Ahmed. In *The Cultural Politics of Emotion*, Ahmed (2004) theorizes emotion, a complex and contested concept in the affect theory field. She characterizes emotions as intentional, insofar as "they are 'about' something: they involve a direction or orientation towards an object" (7). Ahmed argues that emotion as affective force orients, mobilizes, and moves those who feel it in the direction of the emotion's object. So rather than materializing within the boundaries of the human body, emotion "arises in the midst of an in-between-ness" (Seigworth and Gregg 2010, 1). This affect circulates and transmits, rippling along and pounding against the surfaces of subjectivities, and it is through this relationality that subjectivities are bound together, and defined against one another. In Ahmed's (2004) words: "It is through emotions, or how we respond to objects and others, that surfaces or boundaries are made" (10). She invokes the metaphor of an economy: a marketplace wherein currencies of hatred and happiness are distributed and invested (Zembylas 2007).

In affective economies, hatred may not be one singular emotion, but rather a constellation of negative emotions including disdain, fear, and disgust. What these emotions hold in common is how they are oriented, and what they do. In "The Organization of Hate," Ahmed (2001) describes the movement of hatred, suggesting that the "sideways, forwards and backwards movement of emotions such as hate is not contained within the contours of a subject, but moves across or between subjects, objects, signs and others" (348). Hate organizes communities and ideologies—online comment boards, political constituencies, peer groups, communities of experts—by moving through and herding together subjects with a common collection of negative orientations, or positionings defined by their "againstness." But hatred also calibrates relationships between subject and object, hater and hated, by firming up or walling off their boundaries within, between, and around bodies. The intention of hatred that binds the hater to the hated is annihilation (Opotow and McClelland 2007).

We present accounts of interview participants who have experienced hatred directed at their fatness in assemblage. Using intersectionality-as-assemblage theory (Rice et al. in press), we explore instances where participants describe becoming objects of hate owing to fatness alongside other aspects to their embodied being. Following queer theorist Jasbir Puar (2007, 2012), we reframe these entanglements through the Deleuzian concept of *assemblage* (Deleuze and Guattari 1988), a term referring to a complex and dynamic arrangement of ideas and material forms that emerge, stabilize, and dissipate through confrontation with knowledges, identifications, and structural conditions. The framing of intersectional identity as an assemblage thus enables us to account for how hatred flows through subjects and relationships. We map a range of expressions or instruments of hatred—how fat hatred has been distributed—in an effort to show that "there are different workings of hate feelings" (Zembylas 2007, 187). Our interest is in exploring how anti-fat sentiment circulates, entangles with other expressions of hatred, and materializes in or as the contours shaping embodied subjects and social relations. We analyze people who experience fatmisia to argue that hatred leaves impressions on them, and shapes their relationships by generating in them shame, isolation, and anxiety.

Mapping fatmisia: data analysis

Through Thick & Thin engaged with how queer folk negotiate, are affected by, and resist body image ideals and body management expectations. We conducted in-depth semistructured interviews with 24 participants residing in Ontario, Canada, whom we recruited using purposive sampling methods. Our data collection methods were intentionally intersectional, designed to ensure that the range of experience captured was diverse. Given the fluidity of bodies and the instability of categories assigned to them, we resisted classifying participants according to weight or size; however, almost all (21) described themselves as being or having been fat. Their chosen size descriptors—ranging from "fat," "big girl," "thick," "chubby," "superfat," "considered big in Asia," "depending," "unsure, curvy, bigger than typical," to "fat but sometimes pass"—begin to unravel how "fat" might be imagined as a relational construct that de/materializes through specific assemblages of bodies, affects, and worlds. Over half also described living with "mental health" issues, which they related to the everyday hostilities directed at them. Finally, almost half identified as racialized or Indigenous using descriptors such as "person of color," "mixed," "Indigenous in India," "Indigenous history, Mayan," "black," "Asian," and "white," demonstrating how race and indigeneity likewise are relational constructs that stick and dissolve across bodies, time, and place. While space limitations prevented us from selecting quotes for this article from all participants, we endeavored to ensure that our findings reflect diversity.

We transcribed and coded interviews using thematic methods (Braun and Clarke 2006) informed by intersectionality-as-assemblage and affect theory. We attended to moments of affective intensity, wherein participants describe becoming objects of disgust, fear, and disdain. Building on the paradigm-shifting work of Kimberlé Crenshaw (1989) on intersectionality, we mobilized the work of scholars who have brought intersectionality into conversation with nonessentialist and dynamic frameworks, notably feminist affect and assemblage theory (Puar 2012). We analyzed participants' descriptions of viscerally charged encounters and embodied experiences of hatred as "intersectional assemblages" or "affective embodiments"—as emotionally charged, fleshy entanglements of fatness with other embodied differences that could not be split off into separate parts. Through thematic coding and data analysis, we identified and organized participants' descriptions of hateful experiences into patterns. This allowed us to map the spaces of fatmisia, or the relational spaces where hatred as an affective force was most powerfully felt: in healthcare contexts, on transit, and while exercising.

Healthcare

According to *Through Thick & Thin* interview participants, fat hatred bubbles up in the patient–practitioner encounter—sometimes subtly, sometimes surreptitiously, sometimes absent words, yet interviewees are clear in their recognition of these happenings as hate incidents. One common instrument of fat hatred to surface in the interviews is presumption, such as when healthcare practitioners assumed participants had or would eventually have diabetes. Leigh, a fat queer cis woman of color with a degenerative physical disability, describes a preoperative surgical consultation with a medical student she had just met: "I [asked] 'If I do go through with the surgery, is there anything I need to do to prepare for it?' And he was like, 'Well, you could start by losing some weight and not getting diabetes.'" The student's response contradicted her surgical team's prior warning that exercising would aggravate her condition in the lead-up to surgery. In another example, Harper, a lesbian cis-femme woman of color who identifies as plus-size and has diabetes, describes an encounter with her endocrinologist's assistant:

"I don't know him from John, he has no record of my medical experiences. Anything like that. And his first suggestion…on how to correct my diabetes is to get a waist band surgery for my stomach. And I'm just like, you don't even know me! You don't know—I'm not obese to the point where I even need to have that done! It's not safe for me to do that! Before you even give me a chance to even look into losing weight the natural way or to try different things, you're suggesting that I go on weight-loss surgery."

Medical practitioners presented to our participants prognoses and recommendations as expressions of concern for their patient or the exercise of their responsibility. Nevertheless, interviewees are quick and firm to juxtapose medical advice against their own medical record: the absence of a diabetes diagnosis, the existing diagnosis of polycystic ovarian syndrome, the necessity of taking medication with weight-gaining side effects, the inability to exercise safely, not qualifying for the recommended surgery. For participants, this common theme of cautioning against diabetes and advocating diabetes prevention via surgical means does not stem from—and even contradicts—their records. The frequency with which advice was given absent evidence was relentless. In Harper's words:

> "It doesn't matter what kind of doctor. It doesn't matter what healthcare professional. Every single time a healthcare professional sees me, there's assumptions about my body. There's assumptions that I don't work out, there's assumptions that all I do is eat. There's assumptions that all I do is overeating when I'm usually under eating. Um, and all of these negative stereotypes that get attached to my body."

Harper is describing the accumulative force of medical assumption. Assumptions about her body get attached, or stick to her. The stickiness of affect (Ahmed 2004; Guattari 1996; Massumi 2002) is one method of circulation, one way in which affect moves. Further, Harper's and Leigh's fatness entangles with brownness in the larger context of a cultural and medical imaginary that racializes fatness and conflates it with diabetes in Indigenous and racialized groups (Fee 2006; Poudrier 2007; Rail and Jette 2015). This alone might embolden healthcare practitioners to make markedly authoritative statements in clinical interactions with racialized persons, statements that impress pathological otherness as natural fact onto fat brown individual and collective bodies. The presumptions that they slip into their encounters with these racialized patients reveal their intention—to expunge fat (brown) life—and with force or repetition, their intention latches onto the patient to leave lasting impressions.

Whereas presumption may be dressed in the guise of medical concern, shame as an amplified expression of hatred thrusts stereotype into a public forum and back onto the racialized fat body. Leigh recounts being publicly shamed in relation to the scale:

> "I was like, 'I don't want to get weighed.' And [the nurse] was like, 'Well, it has to be done before we can give you the MRI.' I said, 'Fine, but I don't want you to tell me what I weigh. I don't want to look at the scale. I'm going to get on it backward.' ...They weighed me. And then he yelled my weight down the hall to the other MRI technicians."

Similarly, Melissa, a queer femme woman of color who describes herself as voluptuous, was shamed in front of other patients at the close of a medical appointment:

> "I remember he had opened the door already, so there were other patients in the other cubicles, and they could hear him. And he said to me, 'You need to lose weight and lower this cholesterol, unless you want to die from a heart attack.' And I was kind of taken aback, because we were done—the appointment was done. …I said, 'You know, it's really inappropriate to say that to me.' And his response was, 'It's the truth.'"

In these examples, the words themselves carry impact, but an intentional component magnifying impact is the forum itself. Here space and audience are mobilized to direct affect by alienating the object of hate from the collective body. If an affective economy does not reside in any one person or thing but is instead dispersed (Ahmed 2001), the space between and around objects can be organized in the service of this economy. If hatred is the emotion in circulation, its affective economy can be arranged to shut out the target of hate, or to throw them out of alignment with the larger body politic (Ahmed 2010). Shaming renders the fat body hypervisible (Gailey 2014) in order to move the shamed to expunge their fat. This has particular resonance for fat racialized and Indigenous subjects who have a tenuous hold on belonging in a country founded on colonial violence and exclusionary immigration practices that still prioritizes white settlers to be its most rightful citizens (Rinaldi et al. 2017).

Finally, another instrument of fat hatred that emerged in interview participants' medical encounters is the refusal to treat. Common across interviews was the medical practitioner's presumption that fat was the source of existing and future medical problems, and that weight loss was the solution—despite overwhelming scientific evidence that long-term, permanent weight loss is not possible for the vast majority of people who attempt it, and that strategies for achieving significant weight loss are more detrimental to all aspects of health than simply remaining fat (Bacon and Aphramor 2011; Gaesser 2009; Robison 2015; Rothblum 2018). The blanket weight-loss panacea—a product of healthist discourses born out of neoliberal notions of personal responsibility for health (Cooper 2016)—pushed responsibility onto the patient, and thus absolved the practitioner of conducting examinations or prescribing treatment. Raine, a Black queer femme woman who is no longer fat, describes her experience seeking help from a doctor when in crisis:

> "There were days when I couldn't get out of my bed. There would be days I couldn't walk up stairs. There would be days that tears would be rolling down my face, because of how painful it was. …And I was going into the doctor feeling quite hopeful about perhaps coming up with some ideas to just work with it, and was just provided with, 'You need to lose weight, that's pretty much it. Get out.' …

I just have a feeling in my gut and in my soul, that this doctor, beyond telling me to lose weight, didn't have much more than that. No specific examples of health issues or reasons why or how to modify things, or a referral anywhere else. Just, you need to stop eating, was basically it."

Vaska, a fat queer white femme woman, offers her own example of alienation. Vaska recounts visiting her practitioner to inquire about a pregnancy test after going three weeks without results. Her doctor instead lectured her about her size: "She pushed back her clipboard and started launching into this speech about how I shouldn't be eating burgers and fries and fettuccini alfredo. And I said, 'I don't.' And she said, 'You must, look at you.'" Vaska reflects on the impact of that conversation in the months that followed:

"In those weeks between blood tests, I had gotten pregnant, and by the time I found out, I was 11 weeks. And…had a really bad diet and was really depressed and was drinking like a fish and in a bad relationship, and I terminated the pregnancy. And I just thought like—my heart was broken. And I realized just how far this alienation from your own body can escalate when we've got these doctors as intermediaries between us and our bodies."

Raine and Vaska describe their doctors letting them down via indifference, or a refusal to engage. Interviewees' experiences align with Ahmed's (2004) characterization of rage against others that "surfaces as a body that stands apart or keeps its distance from others" (4). Fat hatred expressed through acts of distancing still strike a relation, for the affect carries through to impact the fat person. Acts of distancing convey the impression that the fat subject is not worth the effort.

Hate-oriented relationships also do distancing work when they are devoid of care. Drake, who identifies as a Two-Spirit butch woman but no longer identifies as fat, reflects on her experience in the hospital for colon surgery, wherein she encountered a "lack of…human regard." Her friends assisted her with bathing, bathroom use, and bedsheet changes. Drake recalls:

"I had a terrible, terrible vomiting episode, and there was puke everywhere. All over everything. …The maintenance person asked my friend if she would wipe up the vomit. On my food table. My friend said, 'No, I'm not going to do that,' which is the right answer. And they just left it there. They left the room. They mopped the floor and left the puke all over my food table—the table I'm supposed to eat off of."

Drake's experience reflects Sherene Razack's (2015) claim in the context of Indigenous medical care, that "indifference kills": "the pervasiveness of indifference…suggests a shared belief, an understanding that care would be wasted" (112). In an interview with Deborah McPhail (2016), physician Barry Lavallee posits that stereotype—like Razack's invocation of waste—about Indigeneity and fatness coalesce in microaggressions, or violent everyday acts, that medical practitioners enact when they encounter this configuration of embodied difference.

In transit

Interview participants also identify public transit as a site where fatmisia, entangled with other forms of hatred, surfaces. One way hate circulates on public transit is through the perceptions of other transit riders, whose words and gestures impress on participants the need to reduce the space their fat bodies occupy. When boarding transit, many participants describe having to decide between standing up and managing the associated physical pain, or sitting down and managing anxieties over other riders' discomfort with touching their fat. As Harper puts it:

> "Because, in general, there's not any spaces for big women to be around and feel comfortable. I often observe it on the [transit system]…who's going to sit next to who, how's this going to maneuver. The looks that you're going to get if you sit in a spare seat and you're a bigger woman. Being conscious of that."

Vaska notes that while fat riders may choose to contort themselves, the motivation for doing so matters: "I was on the streetcar, and there was a guy sitting next to me, and I was trying my best to just balance on half of the seat. … I didn't want to make him uncomfortable…and I didn't want to disgust him with my presence." Vaska's preoccupation with rousing disgust influences how she inhabits her body: by shrinking away as much as possible, by perching on the seat uncomfortably, she attempts to avoid becoming an object of the affective force of hate.

Some participants—particularly those with compounding identity markers—describe more overt acts of what they perceive to be fatmisia, but which may also entangle with sexism, racism, ableism, and homophobia. Leigh describes public transit as a "fraught space" for her as a fat disabled woman of color. She recounts an experience riding a bus, where teenage boys laughed at her and threw various objects in her direction. She was left feeling the force of hatred organized into expressions of revulsion and acts of humiliation, and wondering what about her generated ridicule. Participants commonly discuss implicit expressions of hatred—inspecting looks, shaking heads, sucking teeth—and wonder whether these gestures are meant to call out their fatness, potentially in combination with other identity markers, among them class, race, sexuality, and gender expression. Anne, a 47-year-old bisexual white cis woman who identifies as plus-size, finds herself questioning whether she is reading others' body language correctly, and whether fat alongside other aspects of her self-presentation inspires hate from strangers on public transit:

"So, I'm not too sure what freaks people. I really don't. It could be the body size. It could be anything…moving slowly over this body. That's sort of—I don't know what it is. It could be everything. It could be one thing. Like I said, something in the eye. But I definitely feel it. I definitely feel something. Sometimes it's a shake of the head. I've actually had clicks of the tongue or sucking on the teeth."

These gestures—disapproving stares, disrespectful headshakes, disdainful noises—become markers of "something," but Anne hesitates to name them as signs of fatmisia. Confusion enters the affective economy to accomplish a form of disavowal—a hegemonic denial that hatred is circulating. Both Leigh and Anne's hesitation or inability to name what inspired their experiences of hate makes sense within the framework of assemblage. Fatmisia in these cases assembles itself within misogyny, ableism, homophobia, and racism to produce feelings of alienation and confusion. Any assemblage of identity markers that moves a body away from the "master code" human template—white, heterosexual, able-bodied, fit, male (Rice 2015)—marks a body as less human (Bahra 2018), increasing risk of experiencing violence. Ahmed (2004) suggests that affective value accumulates via "circulation between objects and signs" (45), meaning that affects like hate grow stronger, perhaps more recognizable to the hated, the longer and more frequently they move around.

Whether explicit or not, participants describe moving through public space with the constant threat of becoming the object of fatmisia. This threat operates in relation to the physical design of public transit spaces, in which small seat sizes, narrow aisles, and truncated gaps between rows of seats impose strict boundaries that rub against the relative out-of-bound–ness of fat bodies. Here, design becomes an instrument of hatred for bodies that exceed imposed boundaries. Participants describe attempting to avoid even greater exposure to the violence of fatmisia by resorting to physical contortion to ensure they do not move into other riders' seat spaces, in an attempt, to borrow from Ahmed (2017) and Nirmal Puwar (2004), to avoid being perceived as "space invaders."

Observing which bodies are permitted to invade space on public transit yields insight into the flows of affects and their relation to power. Vaska notes that when wealthy people and men take up space, they arouse little anger or disdain, inviting instead affirmation, respect, and support, making explicit that comfort is available to those who can afford it and to those who feel entitled to it:

"And it turns out rich people are allowed to be fat. And it turns out that the chairs in first class don't cut into my hips…in first class, it's a lot more comfortable. [Men] are allowed to be big. I remember—I have a friend who's about to be taking a plane ride, and she hasn't taken a plane ride in a long time. And she's anticipating fatphobia, and at one point—you know, she's significantly larger than an airplane seat. But I said to her, if you were a dude, people would be falling all over themselves trying to make you more comfortable, but because you're a woman, they think you're somehow failing at invisibility."

The gendering of space on public transit is captured here when Vaska juxtaposes masculinist practices of taking up space against her and her friend's felt pressures to contort their bodies. Compare cis male entitlement to space to Vaska's experiences, which involve accepting extreme discomfort for the sake of avoiding fatmisia.

While exercising

One of the central sites for the circulation and performance of fatmisia is organized physical activity in spaces like public schools or private gyms. In private gyms especially, Natasha A. Schvey and colleagues (2016) note that fat members are particularly prone to weight stigma, the consequences of which include "negative attitudes toward the gym, maladaptive coping behaviors, weight bias internalization, unhealthy weight control practices, and poorer self-reported physical and emotional health" (10, cited in Ebbeck and Austin 2018, 82). The logic that sustains fatmisia in exercise contexts is that fat bodies are constructed as always already out of place while exercising—a contradiction in terms. Fat bodies are coded as inactive in the fatphobic imagination, a code that situates active thin bodies legitimately *in place*. Fatmisia functions to maintain the physical boundaries of fitness spaces, excluding fat bodies through both overt violence that discourages their entrance, and the messaging and logics that assume fat to be a consequence of inactivity and immoral health choices. Anti-fat discourses claim that if fat bodies knew how to exercise legitimately, they would already be thin. Exercise facilities, then, take on a double purpose: they function both to exclude and to prevent the existence of fat bodies.

The spatialization of inclusion and exclusion in our data cannot be divorced from the settler colonial context in which this research was conducted. Settler colonialism, as a sociopolitical and economic system of racialized violence, is organized around the appropriation of space and the naturalization of the violence that enables appropriation to take place (Green 2014). Within our mapping of fatmisia in exercise spaces, we encounter dynamics that signal long-standing traditions of place-making in Canada that rely on discourses of cultural annihilation in the interests of self-improvement in order for marginalized bodies to find themselves in place.

The spatialized logic at stake in exercise facilities maintains that fat bodies belong only if they are atoning for their size by actively working to reduce it. Fatmisia circulates in fitness spaces to limit the social participation of fat bodies to a temporary role as bodies in transition. Fat bodies are imagined to be shrinkable, and once they become thin, their belonging within the space of the gym will no longer be contingent. Weight-loss messaging, the presence of medical grade scales, personal training questionnaires that require the declaration of a "fitness goal" or "goal weight," combined with ritualized body measurement practices, collude to structure the space of organized fitness as a site of aspirational thinness. Within fitness spaces, fat bodies are prevented from social participation. Consequently, participants describe ongoing internal conflicts as they confront fatmisia in gyms. Exercising for exercise's sake is impossible in the face of persistent fatmisia. As Emery, a cis femme queer white woman says, "it's like a constant struggle to keep it being about [exercise] and not being about anxiety about losing weight. … I feel so awkward. And I feel very out of place. And uneasy. And I don't want to be there because I want to lose weight." For Emery, her out-of-place–ness is matched by internal conflicts about the reason behind the impulse to exercise. She offers:

> "It's much more an internal dialogue and it's much more a struggle within myself like 'Am I really here—I don't want to be—am I here because I'm unhappy with my body, because that feels shitty. Am I here because I'm happy with my body and feel good moving in it? That feels good.' And then I'll be like 'I don't want to do that anymore. It's making me feel shitty about myself,' so I'll stop going to the gym for months."

The net result for Emery is that, because of the weight-loss messaging, alongside spatial mechanisms that exclude non-normative bodies, she simply does not go to the gym. Her recurring feeling that she does not "fit in" at the gym speaks to the power of fatmisia as a place-making device, rendering gyms as sites of curated participation and overt exclusion.

Exercise as the exclusive purview of thin bodies is a recurring theme for many participants. Leigh describes being singled out in elementary school by a teacher who anticipated her inability to complete an activity in physical education (PE) class:

> "When I was in um, grade 5…we had a PE class, and they were doing like, a big run around the parking lot and the school. …And I remember we had a new gym teacher. …He said in front of the whole class, which was about 25 or 30 kids, 'I want everyone to do this run except for [participant] and [friend]'—who was also fat—'They can walk.' And I was like, 'Why are you saying that we can walk when everyone else has to run?' And in front of the whole class he was like, 'I know you won't be able to run the whole way. Because you're obese.' In front of the whole class. And I just wanted to die."

Leigh's anecdote points to fatmisia as a tool of distinction and exclusion. Her body was singled out from the class as abnormal and incapable. Her teacher used the pathologizing term *obese* to describe her, justifying his exclusion of her public participation under the banner of health. Further, Leigh notes, "I remember feeling so ashamed that I was stopping and walking, but then, kids all around me were stopping and walking, because it was such a long run to ask kids to do in the first place!" Therefore, Leigh was excluded from not only full social participation, but also having her exhaustion normalized. Leigh's need to walk was not interpreted as a result of the assignment being unattainable, but rather because of her size, whereas other classmates were able to not have their exhaustion pathologized. Canadian schools have a long history of enacting violence on the bodies of students, particularly using phenotypic distinction as a method for naturalizing violences on the basis of race, indigeneity, gender, disability, and fat (Rice 2007, 2014). Imposing a standardized physical requirement on students and then labeling those who fail to meet it as unworthy is a productive act, producing and inciting feelings of shame, loneliness, and self-hatred.

The index of hatred here is reflected in Leigh's reaction to her teacher's words: she wanted to die. Here, fatmisia materializes as shame in Leigh for being constructed as different, despite the fact that her classmates were just as exhausted from the exercise as she was. The teacher's assumptions about Leigh's physical stamina indicated an interest in erasing fat life. Leigh's reaction—wanting to die—points to its operation, and highlights its goal: fat death.

Conclusion

We sought to map how fatmisia encompasses a constellation of emotions, among them fear, revulsion, disgust, and disdain. Fat hatred was also shown to materialize in a range of expressions, including presumptuous advice, disapproving gestures, open humiliation, and violent words and acts. The frequency and intensity of participants' experience of hatred were contingent and compounded, hatred against fat tangled in hatred against myriad other body markers, including race, indigeneity, gender, gender identity and expression, ability, and class. What holds together these experiences is the driving purpose to the affect, for fat hatred can be shown in all these instances to organize subjects and spaces with the purpose of excluding, expunging, and ending non-normative living entangled with fatness.

The impacts of such an economy of fat hatred, arranged and directed in assemblage with other forms of hatred, are borne out on the hated. Our interview participants recount internalizing anxiety and shame, feeling out of place and like they do not belong, and avoiding public engagement and open confrontation at the risk of their own personal isolation or discomfort. We committed to presenting their experiences as accounts of hatred—so in the strongest possible terms—in order to flag how serious, how visceral, the negative feelings about fat circulating in public space can be, and how deeply those feelings impact their intended targets.

Disclosure statement

No potential conflict of interest was reported by the authors.

Funding

This project was funded by Women's College Hospital's Women's XChange $15K Challenge large-scale grant program with additional cash and in-kind support provided by Re•Vision: The Centre for Art and Social Justice. Our research team represents community partners Rainbow Health Ontario and the Re•Vision Centre; as well as the following institutions: the University of Ontario Institute of Technology, the University of Guelph, Ryerson University, Trent University, the University of Manitoba, York University, and the Centre for Addiction and Mental Health.

References

Ahmed, S. 2001. "The Organization of Hate." *Law & Critique* 12:345–65. doi:10.1023/A:1013728103073.

Ahmed, S. 2004. *The Cultural Politics of Emotion*. New York: Routledge.

Ahmed, S. 2010. "Happy Objects." In *The Affect Theory Reader*, edited by M. Gregg and G. J. Seigworth, 29–51. Durham: Duke University Press.

Ahmed, S. 2017. *Living a Feminist Life*. Durham: Duke University Press.

Bacon, L., and L. Aphramor. 2011. "Weight Science: Evaluating the Evidence for a Paradigm Shift." *Nutrition Journal* 10 (9):1–13.

Bahra, R.A. 2018. ""You Can Only Be Happy if You're Thin!" Normalcy, Happiness, and the Lacking Body." *Fat Studies* 7 (2):193–202. doi:10.1080/21604851.2017.1374696.

Braun, V., and V. Clarke. 2006. "Using Thematic Analysis in Psychology." *Qualitative Research in Psychology* 3:77–101. doi:10.1191/1478088706qp063oa.

Cooper, C. 2016. *Fat Activism: A Radical Social Movement*. Bristol: HammerOn Press.

Crenshaw, K. 1989. "Demarginalizing the Intersection of Race and Sex: A Black Feminist Critique of Antidiscrimination Doctrine, Feminist Theory and Antiracist Politics." *University of Chicago Legal Forum* 1989 (1):139–67.

Deleuze, G., and F. Guattari. 1988. *A Thousand Plateaus*. B. Massumi, trans. Minneapolis: University of Minnesota Press.

Ebbeck, V., and S. Austin. 2018. "Burning off the Fat Oppression: Self-Compassion Exercises for Personal Trainers." *Fat Studies* 7 (1):81–92. doi:10.1080/21604851.2017.1360670.

Fee, M. 2006. "Racializing Narratives: Obesity, Diabetes and the "Aboriginal" Thrifty Genotype." *Social Science & Medicine* 62 (12):2988–97. doi:10.1016/j.socscimed.2005.11.062.

Gaesser, G. 2009. "Is "Permanent Weight Loss" an Oxymoron? the Statistics on Weight Loss and the National Weight Control Registry." In *The Fat Studies Reader*, edited by E. Rothblum and S. Solovay, 37–41. New York: New York University Press.

Gailey, J. 2014. *The Hyper(In)Visible Fat Woman: Weight & Gender Discourse in Contemporary Society*. Basingstoke: Palgrave Macmillan.

Green, J. 2014. "From Colonialism to Reconciliation through Indigenous Human Rights." In *Indivisible: Indigenous Human Rights*, edited by J. Green, 18–42. Halifax: Fernwood.

Guattari, F. 1996. "Ritornellos and Existential Affects." In *The Guattari Reader*, edited by G. Genosko, 158–171. London: Blackwell,

Massumi, B. 2002. *Parables for the Virtual: Movement, Affect, Sensation*. Durham: Duke University Press.

McPhail, D. 2016. "Indigenous People's Clinical Encounters with Obesity: A Conversation with Barry Lavallee." In *Obesity in Canada: Critical Perspectives*, edited by J. Ellison, D. McPhail, and W. Mitchinson, 175–85. Toronto: University of Toronto Press.

Opotow, S., and S.I. McClelland. 2007. "The Intensification of Hating: A Theory." *Social Justice Research* 20 (1):69–84. doi:10.1007/s11211-007-0033-0.

Poudrier, J. 2007. "The Geneticization of Aboriginal Diabetes and Obesity: Adding Another Scene to the Story of the Thrifty Gene." *Canadian Review of Sociology* 44 (2):237–61. doi:10.1111/j.1755-618X.2007.tb01136.x.

Puar, J.K. 2007. *Terrorist Assemblages: Homonationalism in Queer Times*. Durham: Duke University Press.

Puar, J.K. 2012. ""I Would Rather Be a Cyborg than a Goddess": Becoming-Intersectional in Assemblage Theory." *PhiloSOPHIA* 2 (1):49–66.

Puwar, N. 2004. *Space Invaders: Race, Gender and Bodies Out of Place*. Oxford: Berg.

Rail, G., and S. Jette. 2015. "Reflections on Biopedagogies And/Of Public Health: On Bio-Others, Rescue Missions, and Social Justice." *Cultural Studies ↔ Critical Methodologies* 15 (5):327–36. doi:10.1177/1532708615611703.

Razack, S.H. 2015. *Dying from Improvement: Inquests and Inquiries into Indigenous Deaths in Custody*. Toronto: University of Toronto Press.

Rice, C. 2007. "Becoming the Fat Girl: Emergence of an Unfit Identity." *Women's Studies International Forum* 30 (2):158–74. doi:10.1016/j.wsif.2007.01.001.

Rice, C. 2014. *Becoming Women: The Embodied Self in Image Culture*. Toronto: UT Press.

Rice, C. 2015. "Rethinking Fat: From Bio- to Body-Becoming Pedagogies." *Cultural Studies ↔ Critical Methodologies* 15 (5):387–97. doi:10.1177/1532708615611720.

Rice, C., K. Pendleton Jiménez, E. Harrison, M. Robinson, J. Rinaldi, A. LaMarre, and J. Andrew. in press. "Bodies at the Intersection: Reconfiguring Intersectionality through Queer Women's Complex Embodiments." *Signs: A Journal of Women in Culture and Society*.

Rinaldi, J., C. Rice, A. LaMarre, D. McPhail, and E. Harrison. 2017. "Fatness and Failing Citizenship." *Somatechnics* 7 (2):218–33. doi:10.3366/soma.2017.0219.

Robison, J. 2015. "The "Last Man Standing" Fallacy or Why It's Not Nice to Play with Denominators." *Fat Studies* 4 (2):208–11. doi:10.1080/21604851.2015.1004152.

Rothblum, E.D. 2018. "Slim Chance for Permanent Weight Loss." *Archives of Scientific Psychology* 6:63–69. doi:10.1037/arc0000043.

Schvey, N. A., T. Sbrocco, J.L. Bakalar, R. Ress, M. Barmine, J. Gorlick, A. Pine, M. Stephens, and M. Tanofsky-Kraff. 2016. "The Experience of Weight Stigma among Gym Members with Overweight and Obesity." *Stigma and Health*. Advanced online publication. doi:10.1037/sah0000062.

Seigworth, G.J., and M. Gregg. 2010. "An Inventory of Shimmers." In *The Affect Theory Reader*, edited by M. Gregg and G.J. Seigworth, 1–28. Durham: Duke University Press.

Zembylas, M. 2007. "The Affective Politics of Hatred: Implications for Education." *Intercultural Education* 18 (3):177–92. doi:10.1080/14675980701463513.

Index

Note: Figures are indicated by italics. Endnotes are indicated by the page number followed by "n" and the endnote number e.g., 20n1 refers to endnote 1 on page 20.

For Product Safety Concerns and Information please contact our EU
representative GPSR@taylorandfrancis.com
Taylor & Francis Verlag GmbH, Kaufingerstraße 24, 80331 München, Germany

www.ingramcontent.com/pod-product-compliance
Lightning Source LLC
Chambersburg PA
CBHW081544220326
41598CB00036B/6553